Praise for *Charge and the Energy Body*

"Anodea Judith's *Charge and the Energy Body* takes you on a beautiful journey through the subtle energies that animate your body. Based on a lifetime of curiosity and creative exploration, it will help you understand your own workings, the forces that propel those you love, and how to stabilize and harmonize the energies within you and beyond you. I recommend it highly."

— **Donna Eden and David Feinstein, Ph.D.,** co-authors of *Energy Medicine* and *The Energies of Love*

"In this landmark book, Anodea Judith further addresses the role of the chakras in personality and our intimate relationships. She advances her original understanding of the energy systems of life and shows us just how we can ride the wave of charge and excitement and embody that aliveness. This journey opens the door to the inner experience of the authentic self, of our relationship to ourselves and to others. Anodea also pays particular attention to the effect that trauma has upon our vital energy centers. She then provides maps to help us move back into life, and to know and achieve what we truly want in life."

— **Peter A. Levine,** author of *Waking the Tiger, Healing Trauma,* and *In an Unspoken Voice*

"Everything is possible. And the key is in your charge and the energy body. When your charge blends with its source, the universal charge, you have arrived home. That power is within your grasp. In her book *Charge and the Energy Body*, Anodea gives us a complete, original, and fresh insight into the possibility of living an orgasmic, ecstatic, and joyful life—physically, emotionally, and spiritually. Read this book, and you'll have the key to Heaven!"

— **Margot Anand,** author of *Love, Sex, and Awakening*

"Anodea takes you step by step through an understanding of your life force, including how to enhance it, balance it, and use it for healing. With her foundational practices, we can become better human beings and agents of positive change."

— **Stephen Dinan,** CEO of The Shift Network, author of *Sacred America, Sacred World*

"Superb addition to the field of energy psychology with deep insights, juicy awarenesses, and creative practices. Well written and energizing to read, with a nice balance of personal stories, case examples, and theories."

— **Michael Mayer, Ph.D.,** author of *Energy Psychology*

T0286169

CHARGE
and the
ENERGY
BODY

Also by Anodea Judith, Ph.D.

Wheels of Life:
The Classic Guide to the Chakra System

Eastern Body, Western Mind:
Psychology and the Chakra System as a Path to the Self

Creating on Purpose:
The Spiritual Technology of Manifesting
Through the Chakras (with Lion Goodman)

Anodea Judith's Chakra Yoga

Chakra Balancing:
A Guide to Healing and Awakening Your Energy Body

Chakras:
Seven Keys to Awakening and Healing the Energy Body*

The Global Heart Awakens:
Humanity's Rite of Passage from the Love of Power to the Power of Love

Contact:
The Yoga of Relationship (with Tara Lynda Guber)

The Sevenfold Journey:
Reclaiming Mind, Body & Spirit Through the Chakras (with Selene Vega)

*Available from Hay House
Please visit:
Hay House USA: www.hayhouse.com®
Hay House Australia: www.hayhouse.com.au
Hay House UK: www.hayhouse.co.uk
Hay House India: www.hayhouse.co.in

The Vital Key to Healing Your Life,
Your Chakras, and Your Relationships

CHARGE

and the

ENERGY
BODY

ANODEA JUDITH

HAY HOUSE LLC
Carlsbad, California • New York City
London • Sydney • New Delhi

Published in the United States by: Hay House LLC: www.hayhouse.com® • *Published in Australia by:* Hay House Australia Pty. Ltd.: www.hayhouse.com.au • *Published in the United Kingdom by:* Hay House UK, Ltd.: www.hayhouse.co.uk • *Published in India by:* Hay House Publishers India: www.hayhouse.co.in

Indexer: Joan D. Shapiro
Cover design: Tricia Breidenthal • *Interior design:* Riann Bender
Illustrations: Shanon Dean

Library of Congress Cataloging-in-Publication Data

Names: Judith, Anodea.
Title: Charge and the energy body : the vital key to healing your life, your chakras, and your relationships / Anodea Judith, Ph.D.
Description: Carlsbad, California : Hay House, Inc., 2018.
Identifiers: LCCN 2017046140 | ISBN 9781401954482 (paperback)
Subjects: LCSH: Energy medicine. | Mind and body. | Healing. | Self-care, Health. | BISAC: BODY, MIND & SPIRIT / Healing / Energy (Chi Kung, Reiki, Polarity). | HEALTH & FITNESS / Alternative Therapies. | HEALTH & FITNESS / Yoga.
Classification: LCC RZ421 .J83 2018 | DDC 615.8/51--dc23 LC record available at https://lccn.loc.gov/2017046140

Tradepaper ISBN: 978-1-4019-5448-2

15   14   13   12   11   10   9   8   7   6
1st edition, April 2018

Printed in the United States of America

This product uses responsibly sourced papers and/or recycled materials. For more information, see www.hayhouse.com.

To my students and clients,
whose courage and vulnerability have
taught me so much about charge.

Contents

Preface

For as long as I can remember, I have pondered the human condition. As a young child, I was fascinated with what makes people tick. I'm sure I was just trying to make sense of the quirky behavior I saw in those around me. I remember hearing my mother gossip about a neurotic neighbor or my crazy aunt, and I wondered why each one of them did what they did. From a child's perspective, adults didn't make a lot of sense, but they sure were interesting. I made them a constant study.

At age twelve, with my older brothers long gone from the house, I became an unwitting therapist for my parents as they went through a messy divorce. Of course I was inadequate to the task, but it certainly increased my passion to understand—and my longing to be able to do something to help heal the ills of the world. While still in high school, I spent my evenings at the local community college studying psychology, as I just couldn't wait to find the answers to my questions. Of course I became a psychology major, studying what they taught back in the early '70s: operant conditioning, statistics, and basic Freudian theory.

I wasn't satisfied.

Fast-forward to four decades of study, master's and doctoral degrees, scores of workshops, my own therapy, and clients too numerous to count. While I've discovered that the more you learn, the more the mysteries deepen, I do think I've found some important pieces to the puzzle.

I was fortunate to discover the chakra system in the mid-'70s as my disenchantment from college sent me into studies of spirituality and comparative religion. Here I found a map that made sense. It was a lens that brought the many levels of human experience into an organized, coherent system, spanning from our basic instincts to our loftiest inspirations.

But the map is not the territory. What is it that *animates* the chakras? Of what are we made? As I studied Bioenergetics, Core Energetics, Formative Psychology, and the profound trauma work of Peter Levine, along with a little quantum physics and chaos theory thrown in, I realized that energy is at the core of everything. But like the air we breathe, we take it for granted. To most people it's invisible.

Over time it has become central to my healing work and in my workshops taught all over the world.

Energy healing and energy psychology are now at the leading edge of modern healing modalities. No longer content to see mental and physical health as separate entities, the ancient practices of acupuncture, Ayurveda, and yoga are having a revival. Combine this with the New Age interest in chakras, auras, and energy fields—not to mention that we now have modern technology for measuring some of these things—and we have the dawning of a new field that combines psychology, medicine, and mysticism.

Just as we didn't know that germs could cause illness before we discovered the microscope, energy blockages and imbalances are inherent in our common problems, even though we may not be able to see them with the naked eye. Whether it's aches and pains, emotional overload, PTSD, or addictive behaviors, along with the various quirks of personality in general, we are learning that *energy*—if not the answer itself—is an essential ingredient to finding these answers.

There are many books and studies now measuring and proving that our bodies have a living matrix of energy. This research, like the technology of the microscope, can produce important knowledge and create credibility to the experience of aliveness that we seek to understand. I commend those who are doing this research and look forward to what it will reveal as it continues.

But while science can answer many questions about how and what, it doesn't always tell us why. Why do we do what we do? Why do we have breakdowns and breakthroughs? What's at the core of spiritual experience? What makes us anxious or depressed? What makes us fall in love or continually avoid it? And what is it we are really seeking as we chew up the planet's resources with our consumptive lifestyle?

This book attempts to answer these questions. It is not trying to prove that energy exists, nor is it trying to measure it, as I will leave others to that task. This is not a scientific study.

It is rather a treatise on how energy works within our inner psychology, how it makes us who we are, how it makes us do what we do, and how it's behind our trials and tribulations. Once you learn about this vital essence that I call *charge*, it becomes as obvious as the nose on your face. Once you learn how to work with it, you have an invaluable key to the integration of mind and body through its underlying matrix of energy.

Whether you're on your own journey to heal yourself, or whether you work with others in some kind of healing modality, embracing the ideas and realities of your "charge" will serve you lifelong. I believe it is an important evolutionary step for ourselves and our species to truly reclaim our life force—as vessels of the Divine and co-creators of an inspiring future.

Anodea Judith
April 2017

part i

CHARGE
BASICS

chapter 1

CHARGE

|||||||||||||||||||||||||||||||||||||||||||||||||||||||||

The Key to Your Life Force

The basic substance of the person is energy.
The movement of energy is life. The freer the
energy movement . . . the more intense the life.

JOHN PIERRAKOS

Pulsing through the whole of nature, animating each and every one of your cells, is a luminous, divine energy. Its radiance shines in the light of the sun and the reflection of the moon. It's found in the teeming life in the sea and the constant buzzing of insects. It beckons the grasses to rise and opens the flowers in spring. All life carries it, depends upon it, and is made from it. Like electricity in a lamp, it is universal, yet it shines through the individuality of each vessel, with an infinite variety of expressions.

Scientists have explored this energy, measuring and quantifying, yet have not pierced the mystery of its essence. Religions have worshipped it, with volumes of scriptures about its meaning, yet its everyday presence is often overlooked. Lovers thrive on it, moving mountains when they discover it, or suffering miserably with its loss.

We seek this energy like water and breath. We define our moods and aspirations by it. We know it when we find it, yet simultaneously fear its potency. Without it our lives become mechanical and meaningless. As our innate life force, it is ultimately free, yet it has been diminished and restricted—even enslaved.

This life force has been known by many names. The yogis call it *prana* and activate it through breath and postures. Acupuncturists call it *chi* or *qi* and balance its movement through a network of pathways called meridians. Martial arts, such as Tai Chi, Qigong, or kung fu, also call it *chi* and learn to cultivate its mastery through years of disciplined practice.

Freud called it *libido* while Wilhelm Reich, one of Freud's contemporaries, called it *orgone energy* and saw it as an underlying healing force that often becomes trapped in body armor and behavior patterns. Energy healers work with its manifestation in the subtle field around the body, called the *aura*, and some have called it *Reiki*. In the *Star Wars* movies, it was simply called *The Force*, a universal principle of intelligence that we can tap into for guidance and harmony.

By whatever name, these words all describe the same thing: *the basic energy that runs through all of life.* In this book, I will refer to this energy under one comprehensive word: *CHARGE*. This word is part of our everyday life, something even the skeptics can relate to—as in *having a charge about something.* It's a word we can use with a child who is excited or scared: "I see you're really charged up about that, aren't you?" It's a term that a therapist can use with her clients without getting mired in esoteric philosophies: "This seems to be a charged issue for you." Yet this common usage does not at all diminish its mystical nature, for the more we learn to cultivate and manage our charge, the more its profound power is revealed.

I like to think of the word *CHARGE* as an acronym for: *Consciousness Having a Really Genuine Experience.*

When charge is running through your system, you know it. You might shake or shiver, laugh or cry, feel excited or scared, but there's no doubt you're experiencing something. You feel the energy coursing through your body. It captures your full attention and fixates your thoughts. You might like the aliveness and exhilaration, or you might feel like jumping out of your skin, but there's no doubt that a genuine experience is taking place.

Blocked or unbalanced charge is real too, and can cause all sorts of problems. It can make you say the wrong things or make it difficult to speak at all. It can keep you awake at night or make it hard to get up in the morning. It can turn against the body, creating diseases like ulcers, heart disease, or even cancer.

The charge of fear can keep you from moving forward in your life. The charge of anger can destroy marriages or even start wars. Lack of charge can lead to depression, while too much charge can make you anxious. A parent's unconscious expression of anger or sexual charge onto a child can cause serious wounding.

On the positive side, charge not only animates us, but also increases sensation, awareness, and aliveness in the body, intensifying our experience. It rules our drives and ambitions and keeps workers motivated and political parties in power. It's the energy behind attraction, and it's what keeps relationships juicy. Charge governs the feeling and expression of emotion.

Appropriate management of charge is essential to be successful in life. But it's also how we experience who we really are—as living, energetic beings, each with our own unique expression of life force. As a central aspect of embodiment, charge lies at the core of many mystical experiences. It gives an experience meaning and makes life worthwhile.

To be healthy, we need a balanced flow of charge moving through the body. We need to be able to generate charge when energy is required, to feel its pulsation and movement when we have it, and to calm it down when we have too much. We need to be able to harness its power to accomplish our goals. But most of all, we need our charge for the deeply human experience of being alive and connecting to one another and to the source of all life.

What Does Charge Feel Like?

Charge has physical sensations. It might feel like the jolt you get from a cup of coffee, or you might feel a gentle warmth when someone gives you a hug. It can be the stimulation from a good conversation or the tingling arousal from someone's touch. It can course through the body like a child's excitement on Christmas morning and give a bride jitters at her wedding. When a touchy subject of politics or religion comes up with relatives, you might feel a charge rise in your belly that makes you immediately tense.

When shaped by emotion, or when there are patterns of wounding or trauma, charge can bring a tightening in your belly that feels like a stone, or it can constrict your throat and make it hard to communicate or even swallow. Its rise can make you suddenly feel hot or turn red with a blush, while its suppression can make you shiver with cold. It can make your legs shaky or create chronic tension in your neck or jaw.

All emotion is accompanied by some degree of charge. Anger is a fiery charge of self-protection that wants to move outward, while sadness is a heavy charge that moves inward. When you're afraid, you can feel your muscles tightening, your mind becoming hypervigilant, or your breath restricted. Perhaps your heart pounds in your chest, your belly turns somersaults, or your jaw is chronically clenched. These bodily symptoms may be triggered by an emotion, but they are fueled by its charge.

In fact, the strength of an emotion is equal to the strength of its charge. Irritation is a small charge, anger is a stronger charge, while rage is a charge so big that it's out of control. We might have a few tears trickle down our cheeks in a sad movie, or we might heave with sobs over the loss of a loved one, depending on how much charge we have on the issue. Just as emotions take on different shapes and expression, so does the charge of emotion have different strengths and characteristics in the body and behavior.

When we visit the memory of a past trauma, we might feel charge as a turbulent movement in our belly or limbs, or we could lock up our charge to the point of numbness. We feel charge in our hearts when we develop a romantic attraction, and this charge can make us fixate our attention on our lover when we need to pay attention at work. We feel an erotic charge when we're sexually aroused.

When we block or suppress an emotion, we simultaneously block its charge, and this diminishes our life force and creates issues in the body, such as pain or disease. But we can also lose precious energy by expressing too much emotion, discharging it onto a friend, a partner, or a hapless child. We will look more deeply into charge and emotions in Chapter 12 and examine charge and relationships in Chapter 24.

Sometimes charge has a more mental aspect. It can bring inspiration or sudden insight, or it can make your mind tumble into chaotic confusion. It can take the form of a nagging inner critic who won't shut up or persistent worry that won't go away, even when you know there's nothing to worry about. Sometimes charge cycles through repetitive thoughts or compulsive urges or the inability to think clearly at all.

Exercise:

Charging Your Hand Chakras

The following exercise will give you a sense of what charge feels like in your hands. It's easy to do and works for about 90 percent of people who try it, though like any exercise, it doesn't work for everyone. It's also a good exercise for opening your hands to greater sensitivity in preparation for doing energy work or bodywork, or simply becoming more aware of subtle energies.

Sit comfortably with a straight spine. Extend your arms directly out in front of you, elbows straight, your hands several inches apart. Open and close your palms, rapidly moving from all the way open to completely closed. Repeat until your hands feel tired, about half a minute or so.

Then separate your hands about two feet, with your palms facing each other. Very slowly bring your palms toward each other, pausing when they are about six to eight inches apart. You should be able to feel a very subtle energy field between your hands and possibly some mild tingling or buzzing in the center of your hands.

If you don't feel this energy right away, extend your arms again and open and close your hands a few more times. Make sure you are opening and closing them *all the way* in each direction, until your hands feel tired. With practice, you can learn to sense this subtle energy.

Is Charge Positive or Negative?

Charge is essentially neutral, but we experience it as positive or negative depending on how it flows through us, especially where emotions are concerned. The charge of fear, for example, can motivate us to take action, or it can paralyze us. Anger can be constructive, if expressed cleanly and assertively, or it can cause great harm. Sexual arousal, while generally pleasant, might not be appropriate in the moment. Or we might be the target of someone else's sexual charge, which can be positive or negative depending on whether we want that. It all depends on the context.

As children, we received charge from our parents, both positive and negative. It may have come through loving and nurturing attention or through yelling and punishment. We may have been a neglected only child, or grew up in a family with many siblings who were noisy and rambunctious. Our parents may have handled their charge well, being effective guardians of our vulnerable childhood, or they may have fallen into imbalances, such as depression, rage, violence, or addictions, in which case we learn to view charge as negative.

As we grew up through childhood, our parents' comments shaped our permission to even *have* that charge, resulting in patterns that still persist as adults. When we're told to sit still and be quiet, or punished for emotional outbursts, we learn to hold back our charge and view what's inside us as negative. We may have done that for so long, we're no longer in touch with our charge. Encouragement or criticism, reception or rejection, shapes how we feel about our own charge and how we express that charge into the world.

Charge may be neutral, but it takes the form that we give it, shaped by our beliefs, emotions, and experience. Essentially, charge will take the form of the pathways established by your emotional and physical habits, which can be positive or negative. If you are relaxed and happy, charge will feel like a basic aliveness or even joy. If you are a person who tends to feel afraid, increased charge is likely to trigger sensations associated with fear, which makes the mind look for something to be afraid of.

As organisms, we can survive only when charge is reasonably balanced. Too little and we can barely move. Too much and we feel like we're ready to burst. To lead a balanced life, we need to manage and balance our life force.

How Does Charge Get Blocked?

As children we are full of charge, yet we have little knowledge of how to manage it in a civilized world of "proper" behavior. In school, we had to keep ourselves still and quiet at a desk when our bodies needed to run around and make noise. Too much charge in a child is difficult for even the most well-meaning parents to handle, and its natural flow is often criticized, shamed, or punished. "What's the matter with you? Why can't you hold still?" (Or: keep quiet, do as you're told, or otherwise fit in the way you're supposed to . . .)

As a result, we learned to contain our charge. We learned to override its insistent urges and feelings, locking the charge into the muscles of the body—even as we are building that body through childhood. Of course, some containment is essential, for if we followed every childish urge of the moment, we couldn't live in a civilized society. But often we learn the lesson of suppression all too well, and our very aliveness is diminished.

Ultimately we need to learn to manage our charge, but not by repressing it or getting rid of it. Instead, we can *harvest that charge into the tissues and subtle channels of the body.* Harvesting means that we get to keep our charge and nourish ourselves with it, sending it into our muscles and cells. Like a battery, we can store it for use later on. We do that by dissolving the habitual blocks we have built against it. That is the work of healing.

What You'll Find in These Pages

This book is all about this vital energy called *Charge.* It describes how it works in terms of your inner experience. You'll learn how to sense it, how to cultivate it, and how to manage it.

It discusses how charge governs behavior and how it gets blocked and unblocked. It looks at the way unwanted charge forms body armor and describes various patterns of that armor, called *character structure*, that govern our behavior and beliefs. It looks at the way trauma influences our charge and the important benefits and precautions in dismantling the charge of post–traumatic stress disorder (PTSD). In Part Five, we will examine charge in relationships and society. And of course, as my previous work would indicate, I discuss the way charge is handled by each of the chakras.

Most of all, this book focuses on how to use charge for psychological, emotional, and spiritual healing and growth. It will teach you how to follow charge in both yourself and others. You will learn ways of managing emotional charge without suppression, with techniques for dissolving blockages. And you will learn how important it is to run charge through your core, with ways to charge and discharge for better balance—emotionally, physically, and spiritually.

If you work with clients as a therapist, coach, energy healer, or bodyworker, you will learn how working with charge can bring about effective and permanent change in your clients. It will give you a new way of working that integrates mind and body for greater wholeness and self-awareness.

Exercises will be given for understanding, following, self-regulating, and directing charge into various parts of the body, through the chakras, or into areas of your life. These exercises can be practiced by yourself, used with clients, or taught in a group setting, such as I do in my workshops. Anyone can learn to sense charge and practice these exercises, but they have particular value for those who work in the helping professions: psychotherapists, marriage counselors, bodyworkers, energy healers, yoga teachers, as well as actors, performers, and those in management positions, where the charge of the group or company must be cultivated and managed appropriately.

While there are many books on energy healing or even measuring this mysterious and profound energy, few tell you how to use this energy in daily life. Fewer still understand how and why it gets blocked or its essential role in the healing process. Others seek to diminish or control it and waste this valuable resource. I dare to suggest in these pages that the balancing and harvesting of charge lies at the root of all permanent healing. It is to this notion—and to reclaiming the full charge of our aliveness—that I dedicate this book.

chapter 2

MIND
and
BODY

||||||||||||||||||||||||||||||||||||||||||

Energy as the Prime Connector

Everything is energy and that's all there is to it.
Match the frequency of the reality you want and you
cannot help but get that reality. It can be no other way.
This is not philosophy. This is physics.

ALBERT EINSTEIN

I once arrived at a speaking engagement fully prepared to present a keynote talk and PowerPoint presentation, only to discover that my laptop battery was dead. In itself, that wasn't surprising, considering the long flight I'd just had. The real problem was that my power cord was missing. It had fallen out of my case while I was on the plane, and I hadn't noticed it until I arrived at the event. It didn't matter that I had the latest model of this laptop or that I had spent countless hours creating my presentation with sophisticated software, honing every last detail. Without the means to send electricity through my computer, all my efforts were in vain. The software and hardware had no way to connect. Electricity was the necessary interface between them.

In the same way, your life force energy or *charge* is the interface between your mind and body. Think of your physical body as your hardware. You have your own particular model—you may be male or female, tall or short, wide or thin. You may have physical "plug-ins" such as a joint replacement in your hip, a pacemaker in your heart, or a pin in your arm from a former injury. That's all part of your hardware, along with your blue eyes or brown, your muscular physique, or your excess weight.

Onto your hardware, enormous amounts of software have been installed—all your conscious and unconscious programming. From the basic instincts that are "hardwired" into your body, to the memories, beliefs, and learning that you have accumulated over a lifetime, including the language you speak and the habits you've developed, this software is stored on your hardware, in the muscles, nerve pathways, and central processing unit of the brain. It may include the innate knowledge of how to ride a bicycle, play a piece on the piano, or speak a foreign language.

Your software also includes your self-concept, your worldview, your religious beliefs, and the thoughts that guide your actions. Much of this programming was installed before you were old enough to notice it—basically from the day you were born, if not earlier. Other parts of your programming came from your fields of study, your trainings, your conscious examination or changes in your beliefs, your chosen spirituality, or your past traumas. Once upon a time you learned to walk; later you learned to drive. Now that those programs are in place, they happen unconsciously.

Most of us are unconsciously run by our programming. None of us escape having it.

Essentially, the programming in your personal software tells your life force energy where to go in your body/hardware and where not to go. Your program may tell you it's not safe to open your mouth (or your heart), and as a result, the charge doesn't flow into your throat or heart very much. Or your programming may tell you to behave a certain way in order to get ahead and that's what you do with your life force—push yourself to exhaustion in a constant attempt to achieve. If you practice yoga, dance, or martial arts, you have consciously programmed your body to move in certain ways, and your teacher's words may echo in your mind as you inwardly rotate your thighs or move through your routines.

Our programs direct our charge. As habits form, the program is reinforced by the charge flowing through it, creating pathways in the brain and nervous system.

You're likely aware of the programming you have consciously chosen—the beliefs you have adopted and the things you have studied—yet most of your programming is happening below the radar of awareness or even counter to your conscious desires. For example, even though you want to appear confident in a job interview, an underlying "program" of insecurity can make you nervous and shaky. You may know exactly how you want to behave with your kids, yet find yourself yelling at them inappropriately. Almost everyone has experienced "deciding" to go on a diet, only to find themselves eating some forbidden goodie the very next day. Still others try to avoid harmful substances, yet the urge of addiction has its own program that overrides their best intentions.

Consequently, if there is too little charge, you might not be able to activate a program that's already there. You may know exactly how to do a particular dance form, but if you're exhausted, you can't perform it until you're recharged. You may know a certain word or phrase, but until you've had your coffee in the morning, you can't think of it.

Many of your programs work together harmoniously. Others take you in different directions or exist in direct opposition to one another. You may have one part of you that really wants to be seen and another part that needs to hide. Consciously you may want to form a relationship, yet you have an unconscious program that says it's not safe to be close to someone or one that believes you're essentially unlovable.

When charge activates conflicting programs, you feel blocked. You may experience confusion, anxiety, numbness, or awkwardness as the body tries to sort out which program to follow. Do I speak up or remain quiet? Do I take action or wait? Charge isn't particularly fussy about what program it follows. It tends to animate any or all relevant programs in a given situation, and this can be very confusing when it happens.

When your charge becomes blocked, it doesn't just go away. Instead, it gets locked up in the body and hidden from awareness. If it's repeatedly activated and blocked at the same time, it can become physical pain. Or you might experience it as fear, confusion, anxiety, or futility. Blocked charge can inhibit your ability to learn something new, and it can keep you stuck in something old.

Eventually, the blocked charge itself becomes normal, and the mind turns its attention elsewhere. All it takes is a small trigger, such as being criticized or left out, to bring all that charge up to the surface again. But when it does, it activates the old programs, creating even more blocks and frustration.

Your Operating System

In this analogy of software, hardware, and electricity, there are a couple more components to consider. What is consciousness? Is it the same as the software? Is it in the hardware? Yes and no. Consciousness is the "user," the one who is operating the whole body/mind complex. My consciousness is capable of stepping back, looking at a program I'm running, and deciding to run something else—just as I can look at my computer, scan a website, and then decide to type in a different search word. Consciousness is capable of creating a program, but it isn't quite the same thing as the program itself. It is the operator of the program.

And what about the "operating system"? Most computers come equipped with an essential piece of software called the *operating system* (or OS), which allows the computer to handle your e-mail, folders, graphics, and music. The OS is a piece of software that "interprets" your commands and makes use of them—basically by sending the electricity to the relevant parts of the hardware that light up the color red or the letter Q on your screen.

The operating system corresponds to our belief system. Beliefs tell us how to operate. If I eat a certain way or practice yoga or meditation, it is because I "believe" that it's good for me. If I treat people a certain way or refrain from stealing apples at the grocery store, it's because that behavior goes with my moral beliefs.

Everything you do is essentially run by your beliefs as the master programs installed onto your hardware. Just as money coming into your bank account gets spent on the things you think are important, when charge comes into your body, it is directed by your beliefs about what is important, which in turn activates your behavior. And of course, your beliefs then interpret your experience, which further reinforces your beliefs, and it goes around and around.

As charge comes through the system, it reinforces the beliefs, behaviors, and patterns that are already there. Think of two people having an argument. As the argument escalates and the charge rises in each person, they each become more entrenched in their own point of view, often less willing to listen to the other. If fear rises when you go to speak in front of a crowd, the charge can make you feel so shaky that you become even more afraid, and you can think of nothing but what might go wrong.

Just as charge is the prime connector between mind and body, it is an essential way of connecting with ourselves. Some people love their anger because it makes them feel alive. When people are intensely grieving a loss, they are very in touch with themselves. Because charge is *Consciousness Having a Really Genuine Experience*, we generally feel more in touch with ourselves, with another, or with life in general when we are running a full charge. When charge arises in the body, the soul is enlivened.

Charge and Psychological Complexes

You've probably heard about someone with a "psychological complex." We might say a friend has an "inferiority" complex, but complexes come in many forms. In fact, they are very complex! You carry complexes into your work life that affect everything you do, for better or worse. You carry complexes into your relationship that mix with those of your partner. Needing to succeed might serve you, but having a complex of fear might get in your way.

Here's the important point: *Charge is the glue of a complex.*

What do I mean by that? A complex is made from a fusion of several things: *past experiences, feelings, beliefs, and behaviors.* For example, someone may have had a *past experience* of violence or punishment when growing up as a child. As a result, she may have frequently *felt* afraid, ashamed, or rejected. A natural *belief* that could arise from this is that "the world isn't safe," or that "there's something wrong with me," or that "people can't be trusted." The resulting *behavior* may be to become overly defensive, to withdraw, or to sabotage success.

These are all components of a complex, fused together by the "glue" of charge. As long as the charge is in place, it will hold all the components of the complex together, so that when one aspect happens (such as a memory or belief), the emotions and behaviors all happen too.

Therapists well know that merely understanding a complex isn't enough to change it. Many is the client who has come to me with a full understanding of how their brother did this to them and their mother did that, resulting in the way they are now, but the understanding wasn't enough to change the complex. That's because the basic charge at the *core* of the complex hasn't been diffused, discharged, or redistributed into new beliefs and emotions. But to do this properly, we need to understand the principles of charging and discharging, which we will discuss in the next chapter.

Reflection Exercise

What kind of complexes are you familiar with in yourself? Begin to tease apart the components by asking the following questions (in any order):

Whenever I feel _____(emotion),
I think that _____(belief).
It makes me want to_____(behavior).
It feels connected to _____(past experience).

Then ask yourself whether you feel charge as you reflect on these questions. Where do you feel that charge in your body? What does it want to do?

Allow yourself to feel the emotions and see if you can move your body in a way that releases some of that charge (take a walk, go for a run, put on music and dance, do yoga).

After the charge is released, consider rearranging the components of your complex toward a more positive belief, emotion, or behavior.

chapter 3

CHARGING
and
DISCHARGING

||||||||||||||||||||||||||||||||||||||||||||||||||||||||||||||||||||||||||||||||||||||||||||

Finding Balance in a
Changing World

*Living organisms can only function when there is
a balance of charge and discharge.*

ALEXANDER LOWEN

Our bodies and lives function best when there is an appropriate balance of charge. Too much and we feel anxious and jittery. Too little and we feel tired and depressed.

To keep that balance, the body naturally charges and discharges. This occurs through everyday activities, such as inhaling and exhaling, eating and sleeping, working and resting. We receive charge from our environment and other people, and we discharge through various activities and expressions. For the most part, this happens by itself, just as it does with breathing or resting.

We can override that basic balance, however, in various ways, consciously or unconsciously. We can push ourselves past our limits to meet a demand at work, and then fall into exhaustion. We can use substances that alter our charge, such as coffee or sedatives. We can engage in behaviors that heighten our charge, such as race-car driving, getting into fights, or gambling. And we can also adjust our charge through various exercises, tapping on acupuncture points or engaging in something fun and exciting.

When the balance of charge is upset, we become *undercharged* or *overcharged*. Under normal conditions, we might release the excess charge with a vigorous workout, a good cry, or some hot sex; or we can restore our exhaustion with a good night's sleep or a few days off. But when we go through extended periods (or even a lifetime) of being overcharged or undercharged, it becomes habitual and can create serious consequences for our health and well-being. Our charge becomes unbalanced or disregulated.

Charging activities are basically anything that brings the charge level to a higher or more intense state. They essentially energize. Charging activities wake us up, increase aliveness and sensation, or heighten awareness, much like drinking coffee on a sleepy morning gives us more energy and makes our mind sharper.

But that's not the only way we get charged up. Whenever we're faced with danger or challenge, our fight-or-flight response gets activated and our body floods with charge. This takes place through the sympathetic nervous system that stimulates a variety of processes in the body to temporarily increase energy. For survival reasons, this is a good thing. It gives us the energy to fight off an attacker or run to safety. But if we can't discharge through fighting or fleeing, we get stuck in a high-charge state.

By contrast, the parasympathetic nervous system, which promotes relaxation, tends to lower charge. Discharging activities usually involve some kind of expression or release, often accompanied by movements that can be subtle, like a fine trembling or nervous twitch, or larger expressions, such as crying or yelling. But as stated above, we can also discharge through more common behaviors, like working, dancing, or singing.

Some activities, however, can either charge or discharge depending on the state you're in when you do them. Meditation, for example, will calm you down if you're anxious or stressed, but it will lift you up if you're tired or depleted. It's also true of walking or doing yoga, though these activities are also influenced by the way you do them. Vigorous yoga is more stimulating than the yin yoga that holds poses for a long time. A conversation can either get you excited or drain the life out of you—depending on the nature of it, as well as the state you're in to begin with. If you're lonely and undercharged, talking with someone can help. If you've been talking all day on the phone at work, you might feel drained by yet another conversation when you get home.

The general principle is that charging activities bring energy from the outside to the inside and from the periphery to the core. Discharging activities move energy from the inside to the outside, and from the core to the periphery.

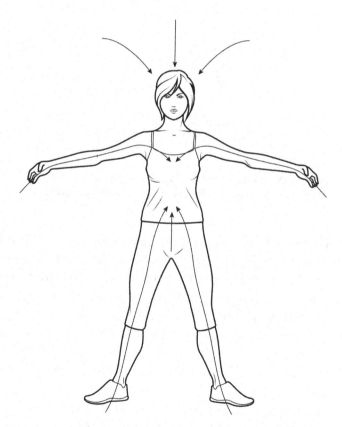

Figure 1a Charging: Charging brings energy from the outside to the inside, through the head, arms, legs, skin, and genitals.

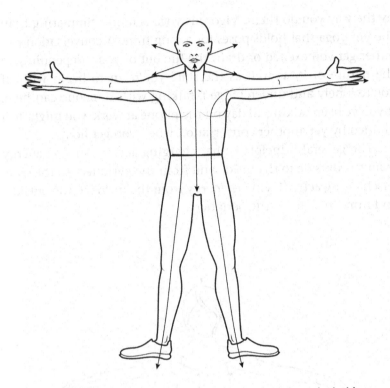

Figure 1b Discharging: Discharging moves energy from the inside
to the outside, through the mouth, legs, arms, and genitals.

When we inhale, we take in air from around us and bring it into the lungs. Eating takes food to the inside of our belly. When we watch TV, go to a concert, or read a book, we are receiving input from outside ourselves and bring it inside. By contrast, when we cry or get angry, we are expressing charge that is bottled up inside and directing it outside. When we take our inner inspiration into creating a work of art, we are moving from inside to outside. When we teach or work hard, we are taking what is within us into an outer expression.

The following is a list of common activities that increase or decrease charge, as well as some that can go in either direction, depending on your state. Notice which ones you often use, whether consciously or unconsciously, to bring your charge up and down.

Common Activities That Are Charging

Charging activities bring energy from the outside to the inside. They stimulate and energize.

- **Inhaling.** Breath is invigorating. Lengthening the inhalation or breathing more rapidly will increase charge in the body. This is why the fight-or-flight response is usually accompanied by faster breathing, which brings more energy to the muscles of the body.

- **Eating.** Food contains calories that can be converted into energy. We eat in order to energize our activities. This isn't always immediate, however, as we often feel sluggish when we eat too much, but at its most basic level, food is energy that comes from outside to inside as fuel for activity.

- **Resting.** We rest in order to recharge. Ideally, we wake up in the morning with more charge than the night before. There are some exceptions, however, as when resting will calm us down from a difficult or stressful day, subtly discharging while we sleep. There are also people who don't sleep deeply and rarely feel rested in the morning. That means they can't go to a low enough charge state to really rest and to be empty enough to fill up again.

- **Sexual arousal.** Visual stimulation, such as a picture in a magazine; flirting with an attractive woman at a party; or engaging in sexual foreplay arouses sexual energy. When aroused, there is a noticeable increase of charge. We have more sensation and an increased awareness of the energy in our body, including desire. As sexual energy builds in the process of lovemaking, charge continues to rise until the point of orgasm, which then discharges that energy.

- **Feeling emotion.** Feeling an emotion usually brings up charge in the body. Feeling the irritation of anger, the contraction of fear, or even the heaviness of grief increases charge in the body. Dread has a charge to it, but so does happiness, anticipation, or elation. Expressing the emotion outwardly would be a discharge, but simply "having" the emotion brings up the charge.

- **Stimulating the senses.** Most stimulation is charging, whether it is touch, music, reading, watching a movie, hearing a loud noise, or seeing a provocative image. This charge may be experienced as positive or negative, depending on the stimulus and whether it's wanted or not. Sexual stimulus from a chosen partner is usually positive, but negative from an intrusive stranger. The beauty of nature may have a positive charge, while an image of violence creates a negative charge.

- **Feeling important.** Just watch someone important enter a room and you can feel the charge around them. Everyone bustles to meet their needs, snaps pictures, or swarms around them. We all get a charge out of feeling important, and some people try to be important in order to feel that charge. In the same way, some experiences stand out as more important than others, such as a wedding or a funeral. These experiences hold more charge than a typical day at work.

- **Finding meaning.** Like importance, the more meaning something has, the more charge it has. The reverse is also true: that which holds more charge carries more meaning. Meaning and charge are intrinsically related. If you lost your wedding ring, it would bring up more charge than losing your water bottle, simply because it holds more meaning.

- **Experiencing memories.** Memories, positive or negative, have a charge. You can feel a warm charge in your heart by thinking of a moment when you felt loved or appreciated. You can feel a charge in your gut remembering a painful incident from your childhood or even something that happened last week. Some memories hold more charge than others.

- **Holding religious beliefs.** Our experience of the Divine—however we perceive that to be—is, among other things, an experience of charge. It has importance, meaning, and emotional overtones, and it is often stimulating. Religious holidays have charge, as do rituals, moral codes, and religious objects. We get filled up and charged up by worship. Religious beliefs carry tremendous charge—enough to fight wars. Consider the energy of religious persecutions or fanaticism, and you see the effects of religious charge at work. However, spiritual charge can also be ecstatic, joyful, and loving. Seeking the charge of spiritual experiences is usually at the foundation of religious practice.

Common Activities That Are Discharging

Discharging is basically anything that moves the charge from the interior of the body to the exterior environment. We discharge through self-expression and creativity, physical and mental activity, and release of emotions. The following are some common ways that discharging occurs:

- **Exhaling.** Exhaling literally moves the breath from the inside to the outside. Slowing the breath, extending the exhales, and breathing from the belly have a calming effect. This increases relaxation and activates the parasympathetic nervous system. Virtually all spoken communication involves exhaling. To block a discharge, one might unconsciously hold their breath.

- **Expressing.** Talking, yelling, screaming, singing, or even writing is usually a discharge. Getting something off your chest helps to discharge the energy of a memory or experience. Releasing the emotion of anger through yelling or hitting is a major discharge, but so is crying (which emphasizes the exhalation), wailing, or even complaining (which is milder). And to repeat this important point: *feeling* an emotion is charging, while *expressing* an emotion is discharging.

- **Engaging in activity.** Most of the things we do expend energy. Exercise, performing, working, cleaning, dancing, or singing generally fall into the category of discharging. While some enjoyable activities may feel like they charge you up, such as dancing or playing music, they will eventually make you tired if you engage in them long enough without a break.

- **Working.** Most work is also a discharge, as it's basically an activity or output. Whether it's grading papers or digging ditches, work requires energy to do it. We spend that energy in making something happen, which is why we feel tired at the end of the day. Even intellectual work can be discharging, though that is a more tricky example, as a full day of sitting at a desk can leave us wanting to do a more vigorous activity as a balance, such as working out at a gym or going for a walk.

- **Sexual orgasm.** As previously mentioned, sexual *arousal* is charging, while the occurrence of *orgasm* is a major discharge. This is why it is common to fall asleep afterward or feel more relaxed and intimate. This discharge generally occurs only after a certain amount of charge has built up through foreplay.

- **Creating.** Creativity, such as writing or painting, is basically a form of expression. While we may feel "charged up" with enjoyment while engaging in creative pursuits, like all discharges, it eventually runs out of steam. We can only write or paint for so long before we need to rest, recharge, or generate new ideas.

Things That Can Either Charge or Discharge

Some things can be charging *or* discharging, depending on the state you're in as you do them. If you are tired or "undercharged" when you engage in these activities, they will leave you more energized. If you are tense or "overcharged," then these things might help you relax.

- **Meditation.** Meditation can bring you toward balance, by simply allowing the charge to regulate. If you're stressed or anxious, meditation can calm you down. If you're tired, meditation can recharge your batteries.

- **Yoga.** The practice of yoga can also take you in either direction of charging and discharging. Like meditation, it can calm you if you're tense and energize you if you're tired. However, it can also depend on the type of yoga: fast, aerobic-type yoga, like an exercise class, can more often be invigorating, at least temporarily, but again, we can only do so much of it before we eventually tire. Slow yoga, such as yin yoga or restorative yoga, where poses are held for a long time, is more likely to leave you relaxed. But even these forms can regulate you in either direction, as, for example, restorative yoga can bring your energy back up when you're tired or depleted, and vigorous yoga can leave you tired.

- **Conversation.** While talking or expressing is generally a discharge, conversation involves both speaking and listening. A good conversation can leave you inspired and charged up, or it can leave you depleted. Conversation about a charged issue can leave you triggered and activated, while getting something off your chest can make you feel calmer. Like most discharges, you can't do it indefinitely. Even conversation can become tiring after a while, as can someone else's constant chatter.

- **Exercise.** While exercise expends energy and is generally a discharge, it can sometimes leave you more energized by conditioning your body and getting your metabolism going. If tired, exercise might bring your energy level up. If you're tense, it might allow you to let off steam.

- **Receiving massage.** While touch is a stimulation that generally brings charge into the body, a relaxing massage can ease stress and bring the charge level down, or it can rejuvenate a tired body. Like yoga, some of this depends on the nature of touch—whether it is soft and soothing or vigorous and intense.

CHARGING	DISCHARGING	EITHER
Inhaling	Exhaling	Meditation
Eating	Working	Yoga
Resting	Creating	Conversation
Sexual arousal	Orgasm	Exercise
Feeling emotion	Expressing emotion	Massage
Stimulation	Activities in general	Walking
Importance	Yelling	Being in nature
Memories	Hitting	
Meaning	Running	
Religion	Giving	

Overcharging and Undercharging

If you are in a job where you're stimulated all day, through constant exposure to noise, phones, arguments, or job pressure, without taking time to discharge, then you become overcharged, a state we call stress. It might be due to a personal block, or it might be due to circumstances, like a demanding period of time with work and kids. Too much charge on the inside makes us feel like we're going to fall apart or burst at the seams. This state is often equated with anxiety.

On the other end of the spectrum, you become depleted if you are giving out more than you're taking in, or if you don't have time to rest and recharge. Now the pressure outside is greater than inside, which makes us feel like we want to collapse and bury our heads under the covers. Without the energy we need, everything feels overwhelming. This can lead to burnout, exhaustion, and depression.

When we can't successfully charge or discharge, or when we spend too much time at either end of the spectrum, we become either "overcharged" or "undercharged." Overcharged people are carrying around too much charge for their body, unable to discharge. Undercharged people are depleted and need to receive energy to recharge.

When these states of imbalanced charge become chronic, we take them as normal. Then they become lodged into the tissues of the body, the behavior, and beliefs, all of which support maintaining this unbalanced state.

We balance our charge through any of the activities listed or through specific exercises you will encounter in this book. We also may need to balance our charge between parts of the body, such as the upper body containing more charge than the lower body, or vice versa. But first we need to reflect on our baseline state and do some assessment.

Reflection Exercise

- Do you consider yourself to be generally a high-charge person or a low-charge person?

- List the charging activities that are natural for you as well as the ways you find yourself discharging. Do you tend to charge more than discharge, or vice versa?

- Is the environment you are typically engaged with highly charged or slow and quiet? What effect does that environment have on you? What is the ratio between the charge you experience on the inside and the charge in your work or home environment?

- What are some of the things you do to regulate your charge under stress?

chapter 4

RIDING
the
WAVE

||||||||||||||||||||||||||||||||||||||||||||

The Charge–Discharge Cycle

The amount of spirit a person has is determined by how alive and vibrant he is, literally by how much energy he has.

ALEXANDER LOWEN

It was 1967. The civil rights movement was raging. In July alone, demonstrations in Detroit left 43 African Americans dead and another 1,200 injured,[1] with another 23 killed in Newark, and $10 million in property damage.[2] Television revealed the ugly truth of oppression, and racial tensions were high.

Meanwhile, out on the edge of a California cliff, in a place called Esalen, the consciousness movement was just getting started. So was the phenomenon of "encounter groups"—people coming together to speak their truth in hopes of breaking through to something real.

George Leonard, a white Southerner, humanistic psychology researcher, and president emeritus of Esalen, had an idea: bring racially diverse groups together in encounter groups and see if it could make a difference. He invited Dr. Price Cobbs, an African

American psychiatrist and author of a book later published called *Black Rage,* to conduct a series of workshop experiments.

The first workshop was called *Racial Confrontation as Transcendental Experience.* Thirty-five people attended, more whites than blacks, as well as some Asians, and more men than women. Most, but not all, were middle-class. It was an intense weekend, beginning Friday night, resuming Saturday at noon, and continuing 24 hours straight through to midday Sunday. They hoped the intensity of the situation, coupled with the stress of exhaustion, would create a breakthrough.

The first evening, the facilitators noticed the conversation was mostly small talk. Various exercises included moving from person to person and stating what they felt about them. Despite setting up rules that encouraged everyone to communicate deeply, with no holds barred, people were not really connecting with one another. Nothing seemed to be getting anywhere.

As the workshop deepened the next day and night, long-held anger and frustration began to come out. But still, the leaders felt that something wasn't working. People were not hearing one another. But eventually, things reached a fever pitch, with everyone yelling and screaming at once. Then something unexpected happened. The group became quieter. They began to laugh. They started listening to each other. They expressed empathy. Some were crying; others were hugging. The breakthrough had occurred.

Leonard, who recorded the sessions, listened to the tapes afterward to understand just what had happened. In his book *The Silent Pulse,* he writes:

> There is a section on one of the tapes that is particularly revealing. It comes around the middle of a marathon and consists of practically everyone in the group talking at once, cursing, shouting, and stamping their feet. Playing this section again and again, I began to hear it, not as words in the usual sense, but as music—a mad, Wagnerian crescendo and diminuendo, having its own internal rhythm, and even a rising and falling pitch. Near the end of the section, some of the shouts and curses began turning into laughter. Then a strange thing happens: the entire

group suddenly stops, then begins again more quietly—all in perfect rhythm. After this, the encounter resumes with a new tone of tenderness and ease. It's as if the pendulums of understanding are swinging together, the heart cells beating as one.[3]

Leonard explains this experience as a phenomenon of rhythmic entrainment—that the different rhythms of white and black speech took time to gel into a common rhythm. That may be true, but I see it another way. It follows the pattern of the charge-discharge cycle, a natural way that charge expresses and balances itself.

In the encounter group, it began with the *stimulation* of diverse people coming together. Even as they engaged in polite conversation, their charge was subconsciously getting triggered. As they "encountered" one another more and more, the charge in each person increased, as did the *tension* in the room. That tension grew until it reached a point of *discharge* (everyone yelling at once), then settled into a new place of *relaxation*, allowing boundaries to dissolve and a new state of connection to occur. This perfectly reflects the following four-stage cycle, though not all situations provide such a predictable pattern.

Four Stages of Charging and Discharging

Not only do we charge and discharge naturally through the course of each day, there are various patterns in how this happens. While there is a typical, or even ideal, way to look at this cycle, in actuality, it's rarely the case. We all bend the rules a little, according to our proclivities, blockages, and needs.

Figure 2a shows how charge and discharge theoretically happen. It begins with some kind of charge-inducing stimulus. In an argument, it might be a thorny subject or someone's tone of voice. In the realm of sexuality, the stimulus might be some flirting or an erotic image, real or imagined, that creates sexual arousal. In a therapy session, a stimulus might be talking about a particular issue, like an unpleasant childhood memory.

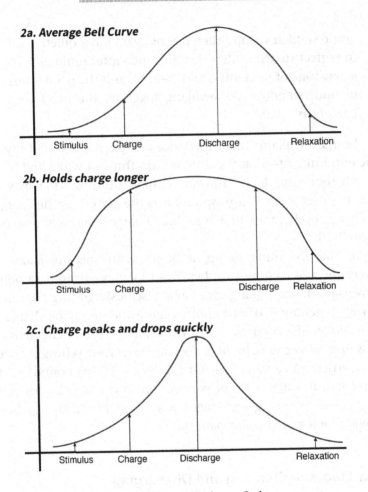

2a. Average Bell Curve

Stimulus   Charge   Discharge   Relaxation

2b. Holds charge longer

Stimulus   Charge   Discharge   Relaxation

2c. Charge peaks and drops quickly

Stimulus   Charge   Discharge   Relaxation

Figure 2 Charge–Discharge Cycle

If you continue to engage with the stimulus, the charge will build. An argument can escalate, with feelings growing more intense and voices getting louder. A caress can lead to a kiss, which can deepen into passion and foreplay. In therapy, one can stay focused on a difficult subject and explore it more deeply, which is likely to bring up deeper emotional charge.

If the charge follows the "normal" cycle, it will build to a state of fullness or peak, and then begin to discharge. The anger erupts into a blowup, or worse, some kind of hitting or violence. In sexuality, the energy releases through orgasm. In a therapy session, it could lead to someone deeply expressing their grief or pounding a pillow to discharge their anger.

When someone is in a *full* discharge, they are riding the wave of the charge, not thinking or inhibiting their actions, which is both the beauty and the danger of a full discharge. This is why we talk about blind rage being so destructive or why a good orgasm can take us to states of ecstasy. A full discharge usually feels like a welcome release in any domain, but it's a moment of surrender, which can be frightening without a certain amount of safety.

The final stage is relaxation. The charge level gently goes down to a state similar to where it was before the cycle began, if not more relaxed and open. In sexuality, this would be the sweetness of cuddling and the intimacy of closeness, followed by falling asleep. After the steam is let off in an argument, two people can hear each other better and relax into forgiveness or friendship. In a therapy session, it is the integration phase that comes after the emotions are discharged, as new feelings and insights begin to take place.

These are just a few examples of the charge–discharge cycle as it takes place over a relatively short period of time. There are also longer cycles, such as working on a project, traveling on vacation, writing a book, or teaching a workshop. In that vein, I try to teach my workshops on this cycle, beginning with something interesting, allowing that interest to deepen, building charge through practices, releasing that charge through additional exercises, and then debriefing for integration.

While the cycle I've just described makes a lovely bell curve, the reality is that it's not always so smooth. The discharge, like the buildup, can be fast or slow. Some people build up charge more quickly and are able to hold the charge longer before they discharge (Figure 2b). Others stay relatively cool and then suddenly "peak" into high charge and release it just as quickly (Figure 2c). This is like a sudden flare-up of anger that's gone as quickly as it arises.

What you see on page 36 are just a few variations of how that curve can become distorted. Many patterns are possible, some of which we will visit later on. But first, let's look at how and why someone might choose to block their charge at any of these four points in the cycle.

Blocking at the Stimulus Stage

Georgina had a high-stress job. She also had three kids at home. Even though she had a good husband and could afford child care, coming home to her kids jumping up and down with the television blaring was just a little too much at the end of a long day. She just couldn't take in any more stimuli. Instead, she poured herself a drink to numb the effects, and that became a longtime habit.

Some people try to block the stimulus to avoid any possibility of increased charge. The Victorian-era prudishness that didn't want to see a woman's ankle is a good case in point, or the Sharia law in the Middle East, which does not allow a woman to show her face, let alone an ankle. Not allowing someone to bring up a certain topic in your presence would be another example. Avoiding situations that make you uncomfortable is a way of avoiding feeling the initial stimulation.

Why would someone want to armor or defend against a stimulus? If there is already too much charge, you can't take in any more until you've had a little quiet time to yourself. If there is past trauma around a particular issue, it might be too frightening to even talk about it, and you don't want it mentioned. Highly sensitive people who hyperreact to light and noise need to block at the level of stimulation. Avoidance is a very common and effective defense.

Blocking at the Tension Stage

Andrew could engage in difficult conversation to a point. But if the charge began to escalate in an argument with his wife, he would cut things off with a statement like: "I'm not going to talk about this. I'm going outside." This was frustrating to his wife, because they could never make it all the way through the cycle to resolution and relaxation. As a result they kept having the same fight over and over again.

Many people are fine with a stimulus, but they can't allow the charge to build. They halt an argument. They flirt but don't engage intimately. They stop a project when the going gets tough, withdrawing from challenge. Or, perhaps, they numb their excitement with a drink or other use of substance.

Why would someone need to keep the charge from building? Perhaps a person is afraid they simply can't handle the charge. There may be too many blocks or too much stress already. There may be a backlog of emotion that is frightening to encounter in its full depths. It might not be the right moment to let the charge increase; maybe the kids haven't gone to bed yet or you're on the job. Or, perhaps, there is a fear of the next stage—discharge—and the best way to avoid it is to keep one's charge from building to a peak.

Blocking at the Discharge Stage

The third stage, after building the charge fullness, is to discharge. This can be a frightening moment because often the ego is not in control and the power of the charge may have a mind of its own. Someone might get on a crying jag and feel like they can't stop. They might go into a blind rage. They might spin out of control and not know what's happening. They might get humiliated, rejected, or criticized. They might feel exposed and vulnerable.

But there is a benevolent side to a full discharge as well. The energetic flow of the core asserts itself, with the body returning to its organic nature. Blocks are removed, and the charge is able to flow freely, without inhibition. We clear out old issues, release long-held feelings. The duality of mind and body become unified as one. We feel whole again. We can genuinely enter the next stage of relaxation—not as an exercise in enforced stillness but as a natural result of peace and well-being. Why do we block at this stage?

If a child were punished for crying or expressing anger, they would grow up to be afraid of their own discharge. If you were in a situation where discharge was inappropriate, such as being at the office, you would have to hold back your expression. You would certainly run out of the room if you thought you were going on a crying jag. While discharge can bring immense relief, it can also be frightening, especially if there is a lot of old stored-up charge that wants to run out the door as soon as it's open.

Blocking at the Relaxation Stage

After a good discharge, we move to the final stage of relaxation, where the charge level slides back down to a low state. This is usually a pleasant state of letting down, relaxing the muscles, being open to change, and renewing one's energy. In a yoga class, it would be entering the pose called *Savasana,* or corpse pose, which is simply lying on one's back, perfectly still, a practice done at the end of each class. In a work cycle, it is relaxing and enjoying the fruits of your labor, without jumping on to the next thing. It can even be as simple as sharing a glass of wine at the end of the day.

It may be more difficult to understand why someone might armor against the relaxation phase. After all, isn't that the payoff that a good discharge brings?

Remember, a full discharge puts the ego temporarily out of control. It's a journey into the unknown. The state of deep relaxation following a discharge can feel very tender and vulnerable. Your guard is down. You're in a state of trust. If there isn't enough safety, one might not be able to relax into it. A child who became a target for someone's anger or sexual advances might feel that being still is just too dangerous. This belief might not be conscious, however, but instead show up as smoking a cigarette, or jumping into the shower right after sex, or rolling up your mat before *Savasana* in a yoga class. It might be discomfort with quiet and stillness or an inability to sleep deeply. It might be moving rapidly on to the next thing, without taking time to savor what you just completed or experienced.

Then we miss the fruits of relaxation. We miss the organic reorganization that takes place as the defense mechanisms and the glue of a complex are released. Without conscious effort, the relaxation that follows discharge puts us back together again in a new and fresh way.

If any of these stages are unconsciously blocked, we are limited in our ability to charge and discharge fully. If we limit the stimuli, we have to control our environment. If we limit the buildup of tension, we can't allow our charge to build into fullness. If we can't discharge, we stay stuck with too much charge and bind it into our muscles. If we can't relax, we can't rest deeply or allow things to change.

Why do we block our charge at any of these points? Because we like to stay in our comfort zone. So that is what we will explore in the next chapter, after reflecting on our own patterns in this four-stage cycle.

Reflection Exercise

- Do you charge up easily and quickly or are you slow to charge?

- Which parts of the cycle do you typically block or avoid and why?

- What is the effect this has on your body? On your relationships?

- Do you try to control yourself or control your environment in order to keep those defenses in place?

- Do you allow yourself a full discharge? If so, do you relax afterward?

chapter 5

the
COMFORT
ZONE

||||||||||||||||||||||||||||||||||||||||||||

Maintenance or Expansion?

If arousal greatly exceeds the regulatory boundaries of the window of tolerance, experience cannot be integrated.

PAT OGDEN

I'm sure you're familiar with what it feels like to be uncomfortable. You might dislike being the center of attention, expressing disagreement, or taking risks. You may be uncomfortable dancing, speaking in front of an audience, or being seen in a bathing suit. Certain people might make you feel uncomfortable just to be around them, and certain topics of conversation might bring up discomfort. When someone has a nervous laugh or clams up in shyness, others can even feel their discomfort. Often clients, when experiencing some kind of resistance, will say that they're uncomfortable with an exercise or talking about a certain subject.

Most often, when someone says, "Sorry, I'm not comfortable with that," we simply let it go. It's become an acceptable way of saying *no*, and it allows people to stay in their comfort zone. Very few people, when they feel uncomfortable, really look to see *what* is making them uncomfortable. Let's look at this on an energy level.

Charge wants to flow freely. When charge moves through the body, it flows through the places that are open and then pushes up against the next block it encounters. If your lower body is free and open, the charge might rise through your belly but then get stuck in your chest or throat. If you're trying to ground, the charge might get stuck in your pelvis or legs. You might feel open in your heart, but your throat gets blocked when you try to express your love.

When charge pushes up against a block, it's very uncomfortable. You'd think we'd all want to release our blocks—that this ought to feel wonderful. Why, then, the discomfort?

Our blocks were put there, once upon a time, for a good reason. Maybe we spoke up and were humiliated for saying something stupid, so we now have a block in our throat. Maybe we were told we were too boisterous or too full of ourselves, and we learned to "rein it in" and make ourselves smaller. Maybe a past lover broke our heart, and we're afraid of the charge of falling in love again, so we block the area around the chest. We may not even be aware of the block until we feel the charge pushing against its edges, bringing it to our attention.

At the same time that we want the block to release, we simultaneously fear its release. When charge pushes up against a block, trying to break through to freedom, all the fears of the original situation begin to arise. Most often, this is unconscious. We no longer remember what we're afraid of; we just have a sensation of fear in our body. We don't remember the details of what caused us to shut down. We simply feel uncomfortable. We don't know what will happen if we release it, and that alone is frightening, to say nothing of having some past memory or experience come back to life. But the more charge we generate, the harder it pushes against the blocks. So we limit the discomfort by blocking our charge—but this also costs us our aliveness.

Releasing the block takes us into the unknown. If we go to a full discharge, as we said in the previous chapter, we are temporarily out of control. The ego is not in charge. Big energies might release, energies we're afraid to feel, energies we think we can't tolerate or manage. That's scary!

And while it's uncomfortable before the block releases, after the release, it can be surprisingly pleasant. We feel free and relaxed, in touch with ourselves in an intimate way. We may even laugh at ourselves, wondering why we were so afraid. We feel relief. It's good to remember in those moments of discomfort that there is light on the other side.

The Sensation of Discomfort

What can be much more fruitful, when discomfort arises, is not to push it away or jump over it but to bring attention to the *sensation*. I will say to my clients, "What is the sensation of that discomfort? Where do you feel it in your body?" Sometimes they look at me quizzically, having no idea what I'm talking about; other times, they are able to pinpoint a physical sensation or perhaps a thought that is related. They might respond with statements like:

"I feel like I want to jump out of my skin."
"My heart is pounding in my chest."
"My palms are sweaty."
"My gut is clenching."
"I feel nervous and jittery."
"I want to run out the door . . . change the conversation . . . not look at you . . ."
"I think you're going to judge me."
"I feel like I'm wrong . . . bad . . . inadequate . . . flawed . . . not ready . . ."
"I feel like I might cry."

In all cases, the charge is pushing at the block, creating a physical sensation and highlighting the beliefs and attitudes associated with the block. Bringing awareness to this edge of your comfort zone is the first step in the healing process. Become curious about the sensation, magnify it or exaggerate it to see what message it might have for you.

In order to track the charge, I might say things like: "What do you notice as you focus on that sensation?" Or, "What happens to your pounding heart when you breathe into your chest?" If it's a thought that emerges, I try to bring it back to the body. "When you have the thought that you're inadequate, what is the sensation in your body?" Or, "What happens in your body when you think you are going to be judged?" If the client has worked with me awhile and is already familiar with the concept of charge, I might simply say, "Do you feel a charge when you say that? If so, where do you feel it?"

Notice that this line of inquiry does not go further into the *content* of the material or situation but rather *follows the sensation of the charge itself.* This is an important point, often overlooked in most talk therapies when someone is describing a difficult situation. We run on about the details and run away from feeling what's going on in the body. We disconnect from the charge and thereby disconnect from a deeper truth trying to emerge.

Where Is Your Comfort Zone?

Each of us has a comfort zone that falls somewhere between having a high charge and having a low charge. Some people are much more comfortable in high-charge situations. They handle stress reasonably well; they can take on challenges; or they might love living on the edge of danger. That's when they feel most alive. If their charge were to drop to a lower level, such a person might feel depressed, vulnerable, or bored. They would be uncomfortable.

Dominic was one of those people. He was a CEO of a large company and attacked his high-stress job with an equivalent amount of charge to meet it. But when he was home with nothing to do, he would become restless, irritable, though he didn't really know why. His mind said he should enjoy watching TV with his wife and kids, but he could barely sit still through a show.

Rachael was just the opposite. She loved time alone, meditating, or just being quiet. She could sit still all day reading a book and preferred to keep things calm around her. Her comfort zone was in the low-charge state. She could never imagine handling a high-stress job or performing onstage. Low-charge people are very relaxed but shy away from challenges. They don't want to rock the boat, because *that* would be uncomfortable. If they are invited to new situations or to high-energy events like parties or crowds, they prefer to stay home.

There isn't anything wrong with either end of the spectrum. It's perfectly all right to have simplicity *or* complexity. Most people consider it simply a matter of preference. They think, "That's just the way I am." But when you allow your comfort zone to define you, you limit your life. You miss out on the benefits of a varied experience. You have to say *no* to lots of things—things that might inspire you, states that might have gifts for you.

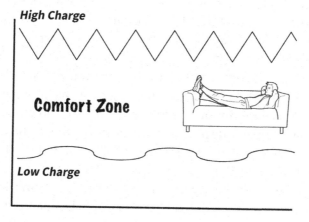

Figure 3 Comfort Zone

Tolerating Higher and Lower States of Charge

Why would we want to be able to sustain higher or lower charge states?

If you can't tolerate the high charge of tension and challenges, you can't handle much responsibility or tackle difficult tasks. It's hard to hold your own in chaotic situations, such as a room full of five-year-olds that just got sugared up on birthday cake, or handling the details of a highly demanding career. You can't really achieve very much, and you might be conflict avoidant, giving in whenever someone makes a demand of you. Challenges bring up charge, and to meet them we need to be able to both tolerate and match that charge.

If you're uncomfortable in a low-charge state, you can't go to deep relaxation. You can't be alone or quiet. You can't sit still enough to have a good meditation. You can't rest deeply, and this has a long-term effect on the body. Patterns are easier to release in a low-charge state, so if you are unable to tolerate that, you remain stuck, unable to let down and surrender to something new.

So you can see that it is beneficial to be able to go to both high- and low-charge states, in order to meet our circumstances appropriately.

Some people have a *wide* comfort zone and easily hold tension, meet demands, and handle challenges, *as well as* experiencing states of deep relaxation or periods of solitude and quiet. Such a person has a greater degree of freedom in his life, as he can be flexible in a wide variety of states and situations, without having to control himself or the environment.

Others have a very narrow comfort zone. They can't handle themselves if there is too much charge, or they feel depressed and lost when there is too little charge. They control themselves and the world around them tightly in order to stay in their narrow comfort zone. They might think everything's okay, but they don't have much freedom.

In order to maintain our comfort zone, we try to stay at the level of charge that we're used to. We engage in activities that are either charging or discharging to keep our charge level within our familiar, comfortable range. This range might not be healthy or expansive, but it feels safe. Too many people narrowly constrict their lives to remain in a narrow comfort zone.

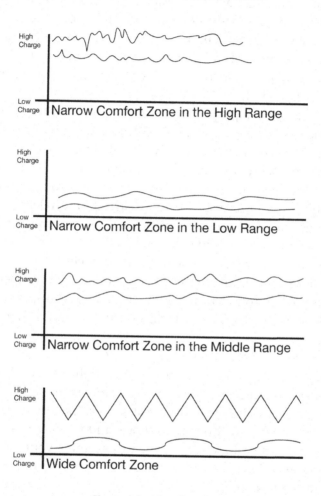

Figure 4 Comfort Zone Variations

Expanding the Comfort Zone

In order to break through to freedom, we need to get beyond our comfort zone. But here's the important point: *Healing happens at the edge of the comfort zone, but not over it.*

In working with charge, it's important to not push someone *beyond* their comfort zone but to *expand* their comfort zone. Pushing beyond it will increase the feelings of discomfort and fear. Then the defenses strengthen, the block is increased, and it leaves a person even more locked up than when they began. Pushing past the comfort zone carries the risk of throwing a person into helplessness, rage, or dissociation.

Take yoga, for example. If James is new to the practice and not very flexible in his lower back and hamstrings, we don't help him by forcing his head all the way down to his knees. That would hurt terribly, probably rip some tendons, and keep him from ever coming back to yoga class again. But over time, through proper yoga practice, the muscles and tendons stretch and release, and James can get his head closer to his knee *without discomfort*. He has expanded his comfort zone on a physical level, and probably a psychological one as well. And he has done it safely.

Expanding your comfort zone gives you more room to operate and allows growth to occur. It creates freedom and dispels fear. You can say, "Wow, I feel okay. I can do this. It's not as hard as I thought."

But *how* do we expand the comfort zone?

You expand your comfort zone by going right to the edge of it and noticing what's there. You bring awareness to the charge pushing up against the block—to what it feels like, to what it's trying to do, to where it's trying to move, and to what wants to be expressed. With that awareness, you can examine your beliefs, release blocked actions, or express emotions, all of which serve to expand the comfort zone.

You can also expand your comfort zone by the Focus and Exaggerate exercise on the next page.

Exercise:

Focus and Exaggerate

When you experience a charge hitting up against a block, begin by noticing what you are unconsciously doing in your body to create that block. You might be tensing your shoulders, holding your breath, clenching your jaw, or tightening your legs. This is what your body is doing on its own, in reaction to the charge.

When you have identified what your body is unconsciously doing, the next step is to bring it more fully into consciousness. *Exaggerate the movement. Make it larger.* If you are collapsing your chest, you might collapse it even further, moving toward curling up in a ball, if that seems like the right expression. If you are holding your breath, hold it even tighter and longer, until you can't do that anymore. If you are shaking your legs or your hands are quivering, shake them even more. By making the movement bigger, it's not only completing the urge, it brings the unconscious movement of the body to conscious awareness.

Take a moment to see what your body might be expressing as you exaggerate your unconscious urge. It might be "Leave me alone" or "I need you." Maybe your body is saying, "I'm all alone and scared," or "I feel like everyone is pushing up against me." Sometimes you might not even know what this movement is saying, and if so, that's fine: simply stay focused on the sensations and urges of the body. If I'm working with a client who doesn't know what her body is saying in the exaggerated position, I might reflect back what it looks like she's saying. "Well, it looks to me like you want to hide . . . push someone away . . . reach out for help . . ."

Slowly begin to relax the exaggeration. By *slow*, I mean *incrementally, glacially* slow, a quarter inch at a time. This allows your brain-body interface to track the change and allows your charge to move to a new place. If you move too quickly, you miss valuable openings that can occur. You also run the risk of not releasing the block. Moving slowly allows the charge to release slowly, meaning it can be better assimilated and—*more comfortable!*

Do not decide with your head where the undoing is going to go. Instead just follow the body's natural process of unfolding. If you are bent over with your hands in a fist, and you *slowly* unclench your fingers, you might find that your body naturally starts to sit upright or your shoulders naturally want to relax. But you are not "deciding" this is the right way to go and then forcing your body to do it. You are instead feeling the natural inclination of the body in its folding and unfolding.

When you reach a stopping place in the unfolding, simply observe where you are now. Spend a few minutes in the new position. Feel what's new. You might experience a warmth or a tingling in some part of your body. You might experience relaxation or clearer vision. You might have a new insight, or you might have feelings come up. Simply be with whatever arises and allow it to move your body.

Anchor that new feeling into your brain and body. Focus on it. What's different about it? What does this new posture or feeling make possible for you? Maybe there's a new belief, a new feeling, a new state of being. Sometimes things do not release in one try. Then you might tighten and release a few more times, just remember to do it very slowly.

Other times, when you relax one thing that you've been doing, another unconscious movement pops up. You might release your shoulders, and then discover that your jaw is tight. Then simply do the same exaggeration and slow release with the jaw. After that releases, return to the shoulders or whatever pops up next.[1]

chapter 6

BINDING
the
CHARGE

||||||||||||||||||||||||||||||||||||||||||||||||||||||||

How We Create Blocks

*Control, due to any habitual restraint on the flow of energy,
is not self-possession but self-imprisonment.*

JOHN PIERRAKOS

Charlene sat in front of me, streaming with charge, but her body didn't move. A few tears ran down her face, but her voice didn't break into a sob. I could tell her self-control was winning out. Her body sat rigidly upright, her hands folded tightly in her lap, her knees drawn together.

Charlene was the youngest of five children, growing up in a highly emotional family with modest means. Her father ran the family like a tight ship with rigid rules. He was of the old school, where males dominated, and Charlene was not allowed to speak until she had been spoken to. She certainly could never talk back, no matter how unfair it seemed, for example, that she had to wait until her brothers had eaten before she could take her meal.

All around her, the family was volatile. Her brothers would tease her ruthlessly as the youngest upstart in the family. When her father wasn't around, her mother would yell, discharging onto her daughter. In order to survive, Charlene had to contain a huge amount of charge. She created a large body in order to do so, putting on weight she couldn't seem to lose, despite numerous diets. She complained of aches and pains. Even though she now desperately wanted release from her blocks, her charge was *bound* into her tissues and wouldn't easily budge.

We have seen how health requires a balance of charging and discharging. We have also seen ways, both positive and negative, that this can occur, and how we might block at different points in the charge–discharge cycle in order to remain in our comfort zone. Now we look at what happens to the body and mind over the long term when the natural cycle of charging and discharging is distorted.

Charge arises for the purpose of action. Ideally, when you're in a situation that brings up your charge, you can use it to deal with the demands of the moment. You can speak up, you can run away, you can handle the crisis—in other words, you can "take charge."

The trouble is, action is not always possible. Children, who are too little to defend themselves, may learn that if they fight back, they get punished further. There might be no place for them to run and find safety. Or they might be told, "Stop your crying, or I'll give you something to cry about." Then they learn that releasing their charge has unwanted, and often serious, consequences—sometimes serious enough to feel life-threatening to a small child.

But what does a child do with their charge in such circumstances? It doesn't just go away. Instead the child (or an adult in a similar situation) must find a way to *bind the charge*. Binding is like wrapping sticky tape around a package so nothing can get loose. Binding ties up the charge in the muscles and organs of the body, creating chronic tension, or what we call a *block*. It can also alter the autonomic nervous system by slowing digestion or inhibiting breathing. It can stimulate the sympathetic nervous system by speeding up the heart rate or elevating blood pressure.

You can also bind charge into a behavior or habit, such as biting your nails, tapping your foot, clenching your jaw, or engaging in obsessive-compulsive hand washing. Binding the charge can lead to repetitive thinking—loops of the mind that may lead nowhere or the inability to think at all. And finally, charge can be bound into addictions, such as overeating, drinking, smoking, or other self-destructive behaviors.

Whatever the pattern, bound charge is less available. It's like having your money tied up in a frozen account and not being able to draw it out when you need to. It's there, but it takes some time to unwind.

Once these binding patterns become established, increasing the charge is likely to strengthen them. If you tend to overeat, additional stress will make you eat even more, despite your best intentions. If you smoke cigarettes, you'll smoke more heavily under emotional stress or the pressure of a deadline. If you have repetitive thoughts of self-criticism, you can rest assured that the charge of making a big presentation will mercilessly energize your inner critic. Increased charge tends to strengthen the defenses against it. This is because we are unconsciously struggling to stay in our comfort zone.

Typically, we bind our charge when discharge is impossible, which means we are *binding a high amount of charge into the body or behavior.* Once bound, it then becomes very difficult to release that charge, because it's all tied up in the tissues. The mind dissociates from the charge and the incident that caused it—and the rest of your psyche goes back to the comfort zone.

However, bound-up charge shrinks the comfort zone. We have less room for ourselves, less freedom to be who we are, and we need more control over our environment.

You can also "flee" from your charge and avoid it entirely, which is a different kind of binding. You might block at the early stages of the charge–discharge cycle and not allow any charge to build, unable to assimilate the charge into your body. This often happens with trauma, where a person is unable to organize their energy in a coherent way. Dissociation can also look like shock, with a person pale and cold after a traumatic injury. Avoiding your charge is disorganizing. It makes it hard to move forward and take care of business.

When avoiding the charge becomes habitual, a person may isolate, have low energy, and remain chronically undercharged or depressed. This is a kind of negative binding, or binding *against* having charge. A person who binds against their charge is trying to keep it out. A person who binds their charge into the muscles and tissues is trying to keep it in.

Overbound and Underbound

Just as we can become overcharged or undercharged, our tendency to bind charge inside or out can create a state of being *overbound or underbound*. This is different from the over- or undercharged state, because we might not feel the charge any longer. Instead it is tied up in the tissues and organs of the body.

Overbinding is a compensation strategy, while underbinding is an avoidant strategy. Overbinding locks a high-charge state into the body, while underbinding keeps us in a low-charge state, not allowing the charge to come in. But whatever we do, these states feel "normal." We think it's just how we are.

Carl was *overbound*. His intense childhood with a raging father taught him to handle a lot of charge. Friends would say he was wound up a little too tight. His children found him too controlling. He was rigid in his body as well as his habits. He worked out at a gym compulsively, and he lived by the rules.

By contrast, his wife, Karla, had an alcoholic mother who was basically unavailable, so she didn't receive a lot of energy growing up. Karla's body was chronically *underbound*. Her body looks frail and tends toward fatigue. Her posture slumps. Her muscles don't hold definition—even when she does work out at the gym. She is easily overwhelmed, and though she doesn't drink, she too is energetically unavailable to her kids—simply because her life force energy is too low to engage with their high energy.

It's also possible for someone to be highly bound in one part of the body, yet not in another. A person might be bound in the chest but loose in the pelvis, or locked up in the hips but openhearted. The legs might be bound with the energy flowing to the head. The heart or throat could be blocked, separating the upper body from the lower.

Below are some common general characteristics of overbound and underbound patterns that you may recognize in yourself or others. Notice there are benefits and drawbacks to each situation, with some traits being at least useful, even if they are part of a defense mechanism. Make a check mark next to the ones that apply to you. Don't be surprised if you have some characteristics in each column.

OVERBOUND	UNDERBOUND
Compensating strategy	Avoidant strategy
High energy	Low energy
Excitable	Calm
Obsessive	Aimless
Controlling	Loose
High metabolism	Slow metabolism
Strict	Lenient
Rigid	Flowing
Muscular	Soft
Stubborn	Yielding
Focused	Lazy

Balancing Inner and Outer Charge

We all know what it's like to go to a high altitude with an unopened bag of potato chips. The bag expands when the air pressure outside is lower. Conversely, if we fill a soft plastic water bottle at the top of the mountain and hike down, the greater pressure at the bottom will press in against the bottle, contracting its edges. (But we probably would have already eaten the potato chips!)

In the same way, if the pressure inside us is higher than the outside environment, the body tends to puff outward, or we feel like we might explode. If the pressure outside is greater than what's inside, we tend to implode or collapse and feel overwhelmed.

Ideally we want our charge to match our surroundings, feeling calm when things are quiet and being able to meet the demands of a high-charge situation when necessary.

Because the charge is always balancing between internal and external states, overbound and underbound types react to outside situations differently. This happens in behavior, emotion, thinking, and body formation. Since the body is a storage battery for charge, these patterns influence how the body forms itself, especially as we grow up through childhood. Aside from genetic inheritance, we swell or shrink, stretch up tall or stay low, expand or collapse, in response to the balance of charge between inside and outside. Let's see what this looks like.

When we encounter outer circumstances that carry high or low charge, we meet them with whatever pattern we have. Any kind of crisis, for example, is a high-charge situation. There is urgency, demand, or danger. Such a high-charge event requires a person to have a fairly high charge to deal with it. Positions of high responsibility and importance both carry a charge and require a charge. Speaking to a large audience has a big charge, and you need to be able to handle that much charge in your body. Making yourself vulnerable or taking risks are high-charge events.

By contrast, situations of loneliness, emptiness, or loss carry a very low charge. We might feel like the wind was knocked out of us. We can get depressed or sluggish with too much emptiness. City dwellers who are used to living in a high-charge environment are often uncomfortable with the low charge of a weekend in the country. Likewise, country dwellers can feel overstimulated on the streets of New York or Las Vegas.

If we then look at what it's like for someone of high charge or low charge to meet various external environments, we see the following patterns.

High charge inside, high-charge situation: My client Jill reported that after being in a car accident with her husband, he kept it together until the police had gone, then suddenly went into an intense rage, which was uncharacteristic for him. He had enough charge to meet the demand—at least for a while—but then the rage was his release. If he had been more tightly bound in that situation, he might have instead become more controlling, manipulative, or dominant. The charge is still there, but the response to it is to become more rigid and controlling of oneself or others.

High charge inside, low-charge situation: Naomi loved to vacation on the beach, but her high-charge husband was anxious and restless. He was used to having a focus for his charge through his work, and in such a relaxed situation he didn't know quite what to do with himself. He felt like he wanted to jump out of his skin. That's because the charge inside was higher than the charge outside, and it wanted to come out somewhere, through his skin if nothing else. When the inside is more charged than the outside, it can create chaos, confusion, obsession, busyness, nervousness, restlessness, and acting-out behaviors.

Low charge inside, high-charge situation: Sandra was a single mother of three with a high-stress job. Without enough downtime to fill up again, she started slipping into depression. She found it hard to think clearly, make decisions, or even clean her house. She didn't want to get out of bed in the morning and face her day. If we don't have enough charge inside to meet the demands of the outside, we feel overwhelmed, inadequate, afraid, insecure, or withdrawn. The pressure from outside can literally cause us to collapse in the chest or belly or collapse in a depression from a weight that seems too big to handle.

Low charge inside, low-charge situation: Kevin was having a hard time adjusting to separating from his wife of 27 years. In their marriage she had been the one with the high charge. She'd created the social situations, she'd gotten things done around the house, and she'd generally kept him charged up with her love and attention. Due to a childhood of neglect, Kevin was a low-charge kind of guy. He didn't initiate very much and was happiest just puttering around in his shop. But with the absence of the outside charge he was accustomed to, combined with the low charge inside himself, he was at a loss. Rather than feeling restless, like Naomi's husband, he felt despondent. Low charge inside and out creates emptiness, boredom, depression, helplessness, or just feeling "lost."

POSSIBLE COMBINATIONS

PERSON	SITUATION	TENDENCY
Overbound	High charge	Tense, obsessive, controlling, angry, overreactive
Underbound	High charge	Overwhelmed, confused, collapsed body
Overbound	Low charge	Restless, nervous, emotional
Underbound	Low charge	Loose, sloppy, unfocused, undisciplined, underactive

Now, when you throw in binding behaviors, you can see that all these combinations create a wide diversity of responses. The high-charge person who can't relax might use alcohol or sedatives to calm down. The low-charge person facing high demand will want more coffee, food, speed, or cocaine. These are all attempts, however useful or harmful, to regulate our charge. Too often we simply blame someone for being irresponsible, obsessive, bossy, or unfocused, without understanding the dynamics of charge that exist within and around them. Often these patterns have been established for decades, left over from childhood strategies that worked reasonably well as a child but work against us in adult situations. Once these patterns become established in our personality, they become lodged into the physical structure of the body in terms of postures, muscular tension, nervous system habits, behaviors, and patterns of thinking. These patterns get lodged into our chakras, become structures of our personality, and play out in relationships. But before we learn all that, let's look at some ways of working with charge in the healing process.

part ii

HEALING

with

CHARGE

chapter 7

BEGIN
in
AWARENESS

||||||||||||||||||||||||||||||||||||||||||||||||||||||||||||||||||||||||||||||||

Tracking and Harvesting the Charge

*Energy is the currency of existence, it radiates from the
deepest centres to well beyond the surface of the body.*

JOHN STIRK

Once you understand the concept of charge, you will begin to
notice it everywhere. You will see it in your colleagues when one
of them gets animated about a new project. You will see it in your
friend when she experiences jealousy or anxiety. You will see it in
your children when they jump up and down with excitement or
suddenly clam up with shyness. You will see it in a crowd as they
swoon over a rock star or a politician. If you are a therapist, you'll
see it in your clients when they talk about a charged issue.

Noticing it in others is the easy part. A person's movements
become more animated. Their voice changes: it becomes louder
and faster, or perhaps even the opposite, suddenly small and quiet.
Obvious signs of aliveness come into the eyes, the breath, and the
body. Emotions come on strong. One might even become shaky,
nervous, or restless. These are all signs of charge.

You can also feel another's charge in your own body, as it is infectious. A co-worker's enthusiasm inspires others in the room. The high charge of anger directed toward us can almost feel like a physical slap, even when there is no violence. Someone in deep grief can make us feel heavy or sad. The excitement of a crowd can draw us into the mob mentality of its beliefs.

What is harder to do is to monitor your own charge. Not because it's so terribly difficult to perceive but because most of us tend to focus on the *circumstances* that are triggering us rather than the charge itself. If you can train yourself to take a pause when you feel activated and put your attention on *tracking your own charge*, then you can make use of this valuable life force energy. *You can learn to harvest the charge.*

Harvesting means you get to feed it into your tissues, absorbing it into your body for the feeling of aliveness and heightened awareness, or for storing it for later use. Farmers, who typically grow more food than they need, store their harvest to use through the winter. What is harvested can be drawn upon, little by little, as needed. It has value. A farmer's worth is determined by the size of his harvest.

Our life force is the most valuable thing we have. We don't want to suppress it, nor do we want to squander it. Ideally, we want to harvest it into our tissues to bring about greater aliveness, sensitivity, and awakening. Like a battery, when the body is well charged, we have energy stored up for future use. We have a wealth of energy within us. In order to harvest our charge, we first have to learn to track it.

Tracking Your Charge

Now that you have a word for charge and understand it conceptually, you can begin to follow it with your awareness. Tracking the charge is a process of observing where it is in your body, what it's trying to do, and noticing what you are doing in response to it. The better you learn to track your charge, the better you will be at handling it, directing it, or harvesting it. You will also create more intimacy with yourself and more skill at navigating difficulties.

You might, for example, suddenly feel a surge of charge when someone says something to you that's emotionally triggering. Maybe the charge is pushing up against your throat or making your gut clench. If you tune in to what the charge is trying to do, you might discover that there is something that wants to be said. Notice what you are doing in response to the charge, such as tightening your shoulders, clenching your jaw, or holding your breath.

To track your own charge, follow these simple steps:

1. *Pause and notice.* Notice when you are activated and take a momentary time-out. Stop the conversation or activity and feel the sensations of your charge. Try to notice as much as you can about it—where it is in your body, whether it feels like pressure or shakiness, emotion, or excitement. Be a curious explorer of this new territory. Notice as much as you can about it, without giving it meaning. Do your best to avoid judgments, and try to be as neutral as possible. Just observe.

2. *Befriend the charge.* Think of your charge as something valuable, rather than something you have to suppress or get rid of. Even if your charge feels uncomfortable or carries anger, sadness, or fear, see the charge as a blessing that is arising within you for your awakening. Separate from the emotion and the story, and embrace the charge itself. Welcome it into your body. It is *your* life force, after all!

3. *Notice the impulse.* Charge arises for a reason—usually for the purpose of some kind of action. Notice the impulse your charge might be activating. You might notice your hands want to clench into fists or they might want to reach for a hug. Maybe your jaw wants to tremble, or you have an urge to run. What is your charge trying *to do*?

4. *Notice how you block the impulse.* Unconsciously, we guard against the charge. We might fear it is too much, that we will lose control, become overwhelmed, or look silly or stupid. The reason is less important than noticing exactly *what* you are doing in your body to block the charge. Are you tightening your belly, holding your breath, or rounding your shoulders? Don't try to push the charge through the block; just observe what you are doing inside yourself because of the charge. As long as we have blocks, charge will push up against them, bringing them to our attention. This is the edge of your comfort zone.

5. *Slowly exaggerate the block.* (See the Focus and Exaggerate Exercise on page 51.) Remember, we don't push ourselves *over* the comfort zone; we *expand* the comfort zone. Pushing yourself will only make the charge more difficult to handle. Instead, slowly *exaggerate* whatever you are doing to create the block, and then slowly relax it, going back and forth between doing it more and doing it less. If you notice your shoulders tighten in reaction to your charge, then tighten them a little more, then a little more. Then slowly dissolve the tightness, following the organic process of your body as it unfolds. *These movements need to be very gradual,* an incrementally slow movement from one state to another. Do this until you feel something shift inside you.

6. *Harvest the charge.* As the block slowly dissolves, allow the charge to flow into new places, without pushing or suppressing. Most often it feels like the spread of warmth, but it could also feel like shivering, tingling, or expansion. It might bring a sense of peace and relaxation. To the best of your ability, allow this charge to permeate your tissues, like water

into a sponge. Enjoy the feelings without trying analyze them.

You can actually try this right now. Think of an issue that brings up some charge for you. Start with something easy. Don't pick your deepest trauma or worst memory. Think of something you saw on TV, a political situation, or an unresolved conversation with someone.

As you imagine this, run through the steps just described, noticing where it is in your body, noticing your reaction to the charge, then exaggerate and slowly dissolve your habitual response to blocking the charge, until you feel a shift.

The more you practice this, the easier it becomes, and the more alive you will feel. Then you can learn to do it in situations where you might feel more charge. It will give you a sense of empowerment to be able to harvest your charge.

Tracking Charge in Others

If you are a therapist, bodyworker, teacher, or coach, you'll be tracking the charge in your clients and students. You can also teach them how to track their own charge, which will serve them lifelong. But be patient. This skill doesn't develop overnight, and this new concept may seem alien to some people.

I begin by educating my clients on the concept of charge. I describe it to them as I have in these pages—a life force that comes through emotions, excitement, and past issues, that is felt as an activation in some part of the body. I tell my client why charge is so valuable and that I will be pointing it out when I see it arise so she can learn to notice it within herself. I also explain that I will help her discover how she blocks her charge and that she can learn to free it up and become more alive and more comfortable in her body. Most people get excited about this new way of thinking.

As you track the charge, here's a list of characteristics that you would look for:

Signs of Charge Arising

- Increased tension in the body—either visually apparent or verbally reported, such as "My belly is tightening into a ball of dread."
- Change in breathing, either faster, slower, or a tendency to hold the breath.
- Change in voice: either louder, talking with increased speed and intensity, or suddenly quieter, or restricted. It may suddenly sound much younger, like a child's voice.
- Tightening of the muscles in the throat and chest.
- Change in skin tone: reddening or becoming pale.
- Sweaty or shaky palms.
- Increased activity in the eyes, possibly darting about, difficulty making eye contact, needing to close the eyes.
- Nervous twitches in the jaw, limbs, or anywhere else in the body.
- Trembling.
- Racing thoughts.
- Difficulty being still.
- Strong emotion.

Working the Charge

Stop and point out your observation of the charge. Say something like, "I notice there's a lot of charge coming into your jaw right now. Can you feel that?" Or, "It looks like there might be a big charge in your chest that is constricting your breathing. Do you notice that?" I strongly suggest stating this gently as an inquiry rather than saying, "You're overcharging your chest right now." This kind of statement takes a person out of their own experience and into thinking there is a right or correct way to be.

If you sense that charge is arising but you can't pinpoint it with your observation, don't worry. Simply ask, "Do you feel any charge when you talk about that issue?" Or if you sense charge is there but you're not sure where it is or what it's doing, ask, "I sense some energy around this issue. Where do you feel that in your body?" These questions help to direct the client's attention and inquiry.

Not all people can answer these questions, of course. Some are so out of touch with their body that they wouldn't feel their charge if it came barreling through at 90 miles an hour. I've seen people shaking like a leaf in the wind who report they feel nothing and can't even tell they are shaking, even though the whole class can see it. But most people can feel at least some kind of sensation, even if it's numbness or emptiness. Through slow and steady work with these sensations, you can eventually unpack and release the charge behind them.

When a client tells me something about his past—maybe he suspects something happened to him as a child, but he's not sure—I inquire as to whether there is charge present when he talks about this. The presence or absence of charge doesn't necessarily indicate whether his memory of the situation is true—but it does tell me if there's work to do in that area. It tells me whether there's resonance with the issue, and if some bit of charge needs to be released or harvested. Whether the story is actually true is not particularly my concern. If it has charge, then it feels true to that person, and that is what I work with. Remember, the story is not as important as the charge itself. The story is about the past. The charge is happening in the present.

Too Much or Too Little Charge

While we ultimately want to learn to harvest the charge, sometimes a person has too much energy moving through the body to be able to do that successfully. Essentially, this means the charge is higher than their comfort zone. And while we ultimately want to expand the comfort zone, it helps to become more comfortable first. To lower the charge to a comfort range, you might need to do some discharging.

If charge is something valuable that we want to harvest into our tissues, then how can you have too much? Charge arises for action, and when the action is blocked, the charge has nowhere to go. It is then stored up in the body, looking for an outlet. It can make you feel restless, jumpy, nervous, worried, sleepless, or like your belly is turning somersaults. Too much charge can feel like anxiety.

When strong emotions come up, they can, at times, seem overwhelming. Deep grief, rage, or terror can be difficult to experience or contain. Yes, feeling the emotions is an important part of healing, but being overwhelmed and out of control is not helpful. And while the emotion itself might not change, the strength of its charge can be diminished, making it easier to endure.

When charge rises above the comfort level, especially when there has been trauma in the past, the body can go into a "lockdown" in order to maintain control. One's thoughts, words, breath, or movements become locked up and unavailable. We "freeze up" and become stiff, hold our breath, or go numb. We can't think straight. Unfortunately, the more charge arises in situations like this, the more extreme the lockdown becomes. This will be discussed more fully in its own chapter on charge and trauma, but for now, take it as a sign that unconscious defenses have taken over because a person is outside their comfort zone.

Signs of Too Much Charge

- Anxiety
- Panic
- Rage
- Overwhelm
- Extreme shaking
- Dissociation
- Difficulty breathing
- Rapid heartbeat
- Difficulty thinking

Ways to Discharge

Discharging moves energy from the core to the periphery. It helps to lower the charge level and return to the comfort zone. Emotions felt in the heart might be expressed through the arms. Fear can move down into the legs. Blocking our throats from speaking keeps what's inside from coming out, so we invite whatever sounds or words want to be expressed.

Under "normal" conditions, a person's high charge will naturally seek an outlet for discharge. Words want to be spoken. Movement wants to happen. Feeling an emotion generally leads to wanting to express it.

There are four main pathways for the body to release charge, as shown in Figure 1b and described on the following pages.

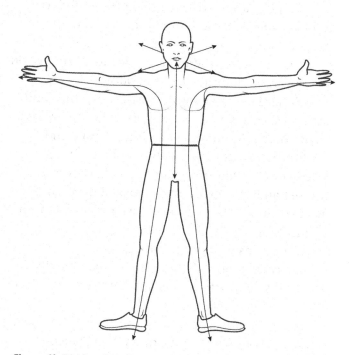

Figure 1b Discharging: Discharging moves energy from the inside to the outside, through the mouth, legs, arms, and genitals.

1. *Downward through the legs and feet.* The fight-or-flight response (which we will discuss more fully in chakra one) energizes the legs. Moving energy downward along this pathway tends to make a person feel more grounded.

   Stamping your feet, running in place, jumping up and down, or kicking your feet into something soft, like a mattress, can awaken this pathway. Often, when a client experiences fear and freezes up, I invite them to simply move their legs as if they are running, even while sitting in a chair. This discharges some of the fear and decreases the flight response.

2. *Out through the arms and hands.* The hands can protect, push away, strike with anger, or reach out to pull someone closer. Any of these impulses can become blocked by past conditioning. Maybe anger was not allowed or there was no one to reach out for, so we learned to override our impulse.

   It's hard to speak without using your arms and hands, especially when you're emotionally charged. To discharge through the hands and arms, find something to push into, such as a wall, the top of a desk, or the arms of a chair. If you have someone whose hands you can push against, allow them to meet you and give you some resistance as you push against them.

   If the arms want to hit, you can punch a pillow or hit a couch with a plastic baseball bat, provided you do it safely, without causing harm to yourself or anything around you.

   If you want to open the arms from the heart, you can reach your hands forward, as if for someone to help you, perhaps a parent, a friend, or a partner. Ask your hands what they want to do and see if you can find a way to safely express it.

3. *Out through the throat.* Using your voice is a prime way to move the energy from inside to outside. Sometimes, just making abstract sounds like a "grrr" or "ahh" can be helpful, and sometimes there are real words that need to be said. Moving downward through the legs or outward through the hands is more effective when accompanied by making sound. Someone who needs to push with her hands to protect herself might find herself saying, "Get out of here. Get back. Leave me alone." Someone who needs to pull another close might say, "I need you. I want you."

Making sound and speaking our truth often goes against cultural conditioning. I begin by encouraging my clients to make any kind of sound that feels natural. Then I ask if there are any words that want to be said. Sometimes I give suggestions, but I always encourage them to find the words that are most true for their experience, changing them as needed. If they are very shy, I invite them to first whisper the words or even just imagine saying them. While this doesn't have quite the same effect, it does move things in the right direction and may open one to more vocalizing once the initial attempts feel safe.

4. *Out through the genitals.* This is one pathway that I don't work with therapeutically, but it bears mention nonetheless, as it is a prime place for discharge. If this channel is blocked, the charge will often be excessive along other pathways, especially the arms and voice. I might give a client assignments to do at home, either alone or with a partner, to facilitate release in this area.

Signs of Too Much Discharge

- Pale skin
- Body slumps or chest collapses
- Unusually tired, lack of energy
- Spacey-ness
- Dulled thinking
- Slow or slurred speech

Of course, some people need no direction to begin discharging. They simply express their emotions, move their body, or speak their mind. If these discharges become too habitual, such as a person who always cries or is always angry, they are better served by learning to contain their charge and eventually harvesting it. The suggestions just mentioned can be used if a person has too much charge to be comfortable, and then must discharge a little before being able to truly harvest their charge. In the next few chapters, we will look at additional ways to deal with too much charge, but first let's look at how to work with the opposite situation: someone whose charge is too low and needs to find ways to increase their charge.

What If You Can't Find the Charge?

When a person tells me they can't feel their charge or when I cannot find or track it in another person, it's either because the charge is too low or because they are dissociated from it. The state of being undercharged can range from tiredness and lethargy to chronic fatigue or depression. It can be a passing phase that might simply mean you didn't sleep well the night before, or it can be a constant struggle to find the energy you need to function.

When charge remains chronically low, it can feel like depression. At the risk of oversimplification, we can say depression results from beliefs in the mind and habits in the body that "de-press" or "press down" against our own energy. Without access to enough charge in the body, it's difficult to take the actions that can better your situation. This inability to "take charge" can then lead to a further hopelessness and despair, which then becomes a self-perpetuating cycle of depression and undercharge.

Signs of Undercharge

- Lack of animation
- Listless movement
- Body temperature drops
- Feeling vacant, empty, or spaced out
- Eyes glazed over, not present
- Generally withdrawn
- Voice hushed
- Tired
- Lack of motivation
- Numb
- Empty

In such cases, you need to increase the charge. Charging brings energy from the periphery to the core or from outside to inside. We get charged up by things we see, hear, and feel as we take them in from our environment. Receiving touch can bring charge into the body. Drawing in more breath on the inhalation brings air from the outside to the inside. Often just doing something new, like going to a museum or getting a change of scenery, can stimulate new brain pathways and bring in more charge. And sometimes, it's just a matter of rest.

Charging needs to be done gradually, while observing our ability to tolerate and harvest the charge. Moving quickly from a state of low charge to high can make it difficult to assimilate and doesn't dissolve the blockages along the way. As always, feeling your body, tracking your own charge, and having the freedom to move about and make sound helps open up pathways to both charging and discharging.

Ways to Increase Charge on Purpose

- Resting
- Eating and digesting
- Reading
- Breath: rapid breathing, focus on increasing the inhalation
- Pushing hands or feet against a wall or floor
- Listening to music
- Receiving healing touch, like massage or Reiki
- Receiving attention from others
- Watching TV or going to a movie

As you practice charging and discharging, you slowly clear out blockages. Discharging old emotional pain can make room for new energy to come in. I know from my years of sitting with clients that after discharging anger, they become softer and more content in their own body. After a good cry, there is an influx of new energy that is light and hopeful.

Energy is infinite as long as the pathways remain open. It is when we close down and restrict the natural process of charging and discharging that we become unbalanced. The more we open the pathways, the easier it is for the natural ebb and flow of that balance to occur.

Owning and Managing Your Core

Moving from the core, from the higher self, therefore, means moving toward fulfillment of our greatest potential.

JOHN PIERRAKOS

Energy emanates into and out from our core. This can be thought of as a column of energy that runs from heaven to earth, through the vertical center of each one of us. Just in the front of the spine. Around that core, like the fruit around an apple core, is the field of our experience. We live in the center of that field, which surrounds us 360 degrees, top to bottom. Some people have bigger fields of energy than others, but we all have a core.

The core is your innate vital self. It is made of universal energy, yet within your core this takes the form of your unique experience and expression. You might say the core is where your divine self resides, as a pure and precious essence. Instinctually, we will do whatever we can to protect this essence.

The core is surrounded by the flesh of the body. The body is capable of sensing both the core and the outer environment and is therefore the mediator between them. It is here that we create layers of defenses, designed to protect the pure essence of the core. If your childhood environment was toxic, you would do whatever was in your power to keep that energy from harming the core. If, on the other hand, you were led to believe that what dwelled within you was toxic, such as a child who is shamed for emotional expression, then the body would use its muscular energy to keep the core energy from coming out. So the body, as mediator, uses muscular contraction to keep energy in and also defensive maneuvers to keep energy out.

These defenses rob the core of some of its energy, even as they try to protect. Our consciousness then gets more caught up in the defenses than in feeling our core, and we lose touch with our vital essence. As the layers of defenses thicken, the inner and outer world become more disconnected, no longer able to exchange energy freely.

The core is not a static thing but a living pulsation of energy moving coherently through the body. When we can identify with this pulsation, we become centered and deeply in touch with our essence. If the body is undefended, that essence is connected to the world around us, with a free flow of energy moving in and out.

The ultimate goal of learning to master your life force is to be able to live in the center of your charge. This means two things:

1. That you stay centered in yourself while running charge through your body

2. That you run the charge through the core of your body

I've had many acronyms for the word *CORE* over the years. John Pierrakos, founder of Core Energetics, calls it the "Center of Right Energy." He states: "No matter what happens on the periphery of a person, the center of right energy strives again and again to reestablish the processes of life."[1] Because consciousness exists at the core (among other places), I have called it "Consciousness Organized in Relation to Energy," and more recently have been using "Coherent Order Realistically Energized." Let's unpack this a bit.

We organize our core in relation to the energy within and around us. We pull away from something toxic to protect our core. We also adjust our core to what's inside us: we hold back our feelings, block our expression, or suppress our charge. We do this with our awareness, then with muscular tension, whether consciously or unconsciously. We say, "I don't want to go there. I don't want to have that. I don't want to feel this. I'm going to block it." Then we disconnect from the central flow of our energy.

What does this look like? You might see someone shift their weight to one foot, tilt their head to the side, or nervously cross their legs, as a way to avoid the full charge coming up through the core. There's nothing wrong with this in the short run. It may be a way of tolerating or managing intense feelings. But in the long run, it can cause pain in the body and blockages in the energy centers of the chakras, which we will discuss in detail in the next section. I suspect it may even be a factor in scoliosis (chronic misalignment in the spine), as children distort their core to get away from something toxic.

Just like a wire, whose copper filaments run through an insulated tube, the most powerful way to move energy is directly through the core. But this involves more than just the torso. Each arm has a core, the legs have cores, each finger and toe has a core, including every cell in your body. What moves in and out through the limbs is organized by the central channel at the core of the torso, in the same way that the spine is the central organizing structure of the skeletal system. When we are well organized at our core, the energy of the whole body becomes more coherent.

As we gain skill with harvesting our charge, we come toward defining CORE as "Coherent Order Realistically Energized." When we work out our blocks, enliven our energy, and manage and identify with the core as a central aspect of self, life becomes more coherent.

While harvesting the charge into our core may be an ultimate goal, it might be necessary to charge or discharge a little to make the charge more manageable, so that we *can* eventually come to live in the center of our charge and have that center be a Coherent Order Realistically Energized. The next chapter will look at some simple techniques for self-regulating your charge.

chapter 8

SELF-REGULATION

||||||||||||||||||||||||||||||||||||||||||||||||||||||||||||||||||||||||||||||||||||||

Tapping the Charge

*Energy medicine is the art and science of fostering physical,
psychological, and spiritual health and vitality.*

DONNA EDEN

One of the more popular methods of dealing with charge falls under the heading of energy psychology (EP), also known as energy medicine. This rapidly growing field regards regulation of energy itself as the medicine for what ails us. If energy is the interface between mind and body (as described in Chapter 2), then it follows that the flow of energy can influence our thoughts and our physical health, just as our thoughts and physical chemistry can influence our energy.

Energy psychology regards emotional, psychological, and physical issues as a disturbance in the energy flow, which then disrupts the optimal functioning of our mind-body system. These disruptions can be addressed through acupuncture meridians, the chakras, the human biofield, and the electromagnetic activity of the body. Treatments can address neurological functions, immunology, electrophysiology, thought patterns, and behaviors.

Energy psychology can be seen as a viable "charge management system" that brings the charge associated with certain experiences back into the comfort zone so they can be better man-aged. As the charge becomes more regulated, a person gains more control over their internal state and is less at the mercy of dysfunc-tional charge patterns. As a result of redirecting the flow of energy, thoughts and behaviors can change also. It's a wonderful tool for working with a wide variety of issues, such as:

- Emotional overload

- Traumatic memories

- Habits and addictions

- Compulsive thinking

- Limiting beliefs

- Anxiety and depression

- Insomnia

- Physical pain

- Allergic reactions

Various modalities are often known by their initials, such as EFT (Emotional Freedom Technique), TFT (Thought Field Ther-apy), and EMDR (Eye Movement Desensitization and Reprocess-ing) being the most popular. Gary Craig developed EFT in the mid-1990s, and by his retirement in 2010, more than a million people from all over the world had downloaded his instruc-tional manual.[1]

There is much documentation and peer-reviewed studies showing the effectiveness of various EP treatments, especially in hard-hit areas like war zones or the sites of natural disasters, where access to long-term psychotherapy or trauma care is nonexistent. Within even a single session, EP practitioners have been able to provide relief or resolution to fears, sleeplessness, negative emo-tions, and other post–traumatic stress symptoms.[2] The Associa-tion for Comprehensive Energy Psychology (ACEP) has catalogued more than 100 research studies, analyses, and articles, which can be accessed on their website at www.energypsych.org/.

Some of the benefits of using these techniques (aside from how rapidly change can occur) is that they can be done anytime, anywhere; cost nothing to administer; involve no drugs, devices, or surgery; are noninvasive; and can be easily and quickly learned by anyone, even children. These techniques work in a majority of cases, and if not, they are at least completely harmless. There is much that can be gained and nothing to lose.

How Does It Work?

The practice of energy psychology utilizes tapping on specific points on the face and body in order to repattern our energetic responses to thoughts, feelings, sensations, memories, and behaviors. As we have learned, any of these things can generate charge in the body—sometimes more than we can handle. They are also the central components of a complex, as described in Chapter 2—a bundle of human responses that are fused together with charge. It makes sense that diffusing the charge would help break apart the complex so we can create a more functional set of behaviors, thoughts, and emotions.

EP manages the flow of charge through accessing points along the meridians identified by Traditional Chinese Medicine (TCM) (Figure 5). While tapping on a specific set of points, one focuses on various thoughts, emotions, or sensations. By regulating the charge along these pathways, the associated thoughts and feelings become neutralized or energized, depending on one's intent.

Meridians are like a charge delivery system. They carry pulses of energy along established pathways the way our highways carry trucks full of goods. If there is an accident or a traffic jam, the flow is interrupted, and some places will not receive the delivery of the goods they need. Over time, those areas can become undernourished (undercharged), while the backed-up energy along the highway becomes excessive (overcharged) in other locations.

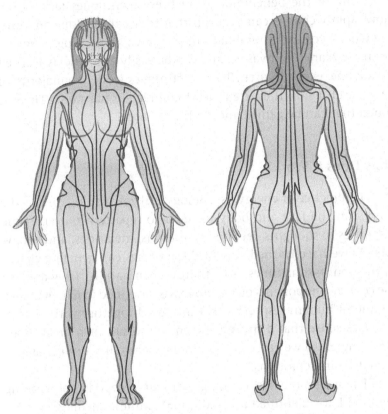

Figure 5 Meridians of Traditional Chinese Medicine

Just like the wires that run hidden behind our walls, with periodic outlets you can plug in to, the meridians can be influenced through hundreds of points all over the body that have been elaborately mapped out by TCM and studied in Asia for thousands of years. Using needles, tapping, or pressure on these points helps to free up the disregulated energy and establish its natural flow once again.

While most people go to an acupuncturist for physical issues, such as pain or illness, energy psychology utilizes these pathways to rewire the neural circuitry of the brain and affect psychological states. If you tap on a pattern of points while you focus on a thought that triggers emotional pain, you can shift your brain's response to that situation. You can also use EP to positively charge more productive thoughts and feelings, such as self-confidence, personal goals, or positive affirmations.

Tapping works on the limbic system, which is a part of the brain that assigns emotional responses to memories, so as to alert us to danger if such a thing were to happen again. But sometimes a past negative experience can be generalized too broadly. Rather than protecting us, it limits us needlessly. For instance, we might have had a hurtful experience with a teacher in grammar school, but that needn't keep us from attending college out of our fear from our past. The amygdala is a part of the brain that processes emotion and typically responds to feelings of threat. When someone is faced with danger, the amygdala is activated and a subsequent flow of high charge is released through the system. This charge has the purpose of handling that danger—either fighting it off or running away from it. It is an inherent biological response to help keep us alive.

When someone has a past trauma, such as a war experience or childhood abuse, the memory alone can trigger a fear response in the amygdala, even decades later when no present danger exists. Visual or sensate cues similar to the original situation, such as seeing a man who resembles the abuser, smelling alcohol on someone's breath, or hearing a sound that resembles gunfire, can trigger the amygdala response, which then floods the body with charge for the purpose of fight or flight. This can be very unpleasant if the man who triggers you is actually a friend or business associate or if the sound that triggers the memory of gunshot is actually the drums in a concert. By deactivating the amygdala, memories and associated cues can be calmed down so that a more normal response can occur.

The Basic Formula

While there are many techniques, the most commonly used comes from Emotional Freedom Technique (EFT), which taps on the points shown in Figure 6, while making various statements relevant to the issue. Tapping is generally done in the order shown by the numbers, and even though some of the points may be paired on each side of the body, tapping on just one side with one hand will usually suffice.

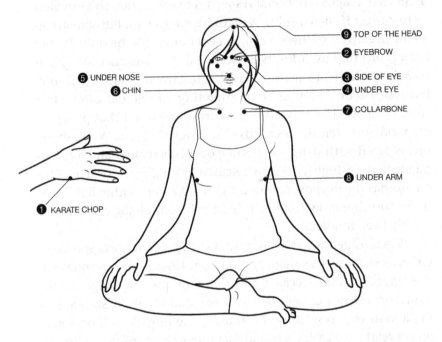

Figure 6 Tapping Sequence: Tap on the points in the order numbered while making your statements. Tapping on one side of the body will suffice.

This is best explained with an example.

Marjorie is just finishing law school and is studying for her bar exam to become an attorney. Unfortunately, she has an intense fear of exams that brings up so much anxiety, she can't think clearly. The mere thought about the exam approaching keeps her sleepless and anxious for weeks in advance, and she's afraid she will fail if she cannot bring her anxiety under control. Marjorie already knows that this fear comes from her father's rage at her inability to solve math problems in high school, but this realization has not yet gotten rid of her fear.

Marjorie starts with an assessment of the problem and assesses the level of activation that goes with it. On this point, Marjorie would say that her anxiety level is about nine on a scale of one to ten, with ten being the highest.

Marjorie begins with a statement of what is occurring, while making positive statements about self-love and acceptance. She says something like, "Even though I am terrified of taking exams, I completely love and accept myself." She repeats this statement while tapping the sequence shown in Figure 6, tapping about seven times firmly on each of the points. By the time she gets to the last acupoint, she can check and see if her anxiety level is reduced or nonexistent. Usually the charge is lowered, if only mildly in the first try. Sometimes it is cleared completely. She then assigns it a new level and might say, "Now it's only a five on the scale of one to ten."

If the charge level is only reduced but not cleared, then she can repeat the tapping sequence again with a statement that reflects how the state is changing. "Even though I have *some* anxiety about taking this exam, I completely love and accept myself." "Even though I don't like exams, I completely love and accept myself." She can then continue to modify her statements until her anxiety is reduced to a manageable or nonexistent level.

Now let's say Marjorie knows that her anxiety is complicated by the memory of her father raging at her while she was trying to do her homework in seventh grade. When she focuses on that memory, her anxiety rises again. This is another component of the memory or complex. She can then go back and tap the sequence again, focusing on her father. "Even though my father's rage terrifies me, I completely love and accept myself," or "Even though my father made me feel stupid and incompetent, I completely love and accept myself." As the charge level reduces, the statement might change to: "Even though my father's presence gives me concern, I still love and accept myself," or "Even though exams are challenging, I still love and accept myself." Eventually, she can make a statement like, "I calmly and confidently take my exam as I completely love and accept myself."

The point here is to fully acknowledge whatever is so, without judgment or denial. When the state that exists is coupled with love and self-acceptance (while tapping), the energy circuits are repatterned. As the charge level decreases, the statements change to match what is, yet they are still connected to love and self-acceptance. If such a statement about acceptance is hard to make or seems untrue, you can modify it accordingly. "I accept that I have these feelings," or "I accept parts of myself," or "I accept that I'm a good person," or for children, "I'm still a great kid."

I myself have used this technique for pain management and found it to be quite effective, at least temporarily. Obviously, it doesn't claim to heal the source of pain, such as an infection or a broken bone, but it can minimize the intensity of reaction to what's going on and alleviate suffering.

It can also help with allergies, as I witnessed firsthand at a dinner of presenters at an Association for Comprehensive Energy Psychology conference several years ago. Lion Goodman, my partner at the time, was enjoying his meal, when he started having an extreme allergic reaction. We knew he was allergic to scale fish, but he hadn't knowingly eaten any fish. However, we found out there was fish sauce in one of the dishes, and that was enough to get him wheezing and gasping for breath. In the past, when this would happen to him, he had to go directly to the hospital, so we were about ready to call an ambulance.

It just so happened that there was a practitioner at the dinner who specialized in using EP for allergies. She began to work with him, using these methods, and immediately his symptoms started to diminish. After the allergic reaction was lowered, the practitioner then worked on the original memory. It turned out that at five years old, Lion had a pet goldfish in a bowl. One day he accidentally knocked over the fishbowl and had to watch the fish struggle and die on the floor. It was his emotional guilt and dismay at the time that produced the allergic reaction, which had continued for the next five decades. Once we worked with this memory and cleared its energetic disturbance, his symptoms completely disappeared for the rest of the evening with no further intervention.

I don't know whether he's dared to eat fish since then, but the response at the time was remarkable and potentially lifesaving.

Pros and Cons of This Method

While its method is simple, tapping can produce immediate, measurable, and sometimes profound results. In situations where the level of charge, intensity of emotion, or severity of symptoms produce debilitating discomfort, the speed and effectiveness of this method makes it invaluable. There are now whole conferences where practitioners come together and expand on these methods, with numerous trainings easily obtained.*

My own caveat about tapping away the charge is that it often does not allow "harvesting" the charge. I'll use the following experience as an example.

When I was working with a new therapist many years ago, the memory of a sexual trauma surfaced for me. Immediately the charge in my body was activated, especially through my hips and thighs. The therapist I was with at the time suggested I do the tapping sequence while I made statements relevant to the memory and accepting myself. Being a dutiful client, I followed the instructions, and within a few minutes the charge level not only came down but was completely gone.

However, this was an area of my body from which I'd felt disconnected much of my life, and I was at least glad to feel the charge in my thighs again. After the tapping, and for months afterward, I had less muscle tone in my inner thighs and a harder time sensing and connecting with them. Because I know how to process charge in my body, my feeling at the time was, "Hey, where'd my charge go? I want that charge back!"

This story does not negate the effectiveness of the tapping techniques but asks for a more nuanced understanding of the charge that people are tapping away. Sometimes a symptom has a message for us. Sitting with the charge for a while brings deeper

---

*   See the Association for Comprehensive Energy Psychology website: http://www.energypsych.org.

insights and leads to other related issues. By allowing the charge to flow freely within the body, we deepen our connection to our soul. The main danger of a simple and effective technique is that it can be used too readily and too often. Discernment is advised.

chapter 9

CHARGE and TRAUMA

If hyperarousal is the nervous system's accelerator, immobility is its brake. When both of these states occur at the same time, a feeling of overwhelming helplessness results.

PETER LEVINE[1]

In my decades of working with clients, I have come to observe the dance of charge with the deepest respect. From excitement to fears, overcharge to undercharge, emotional extremes to numbness, I have seen how the life force creates intricate patterns within each soul. I see how a person's history shapes these patterns and how that shape is then triggered by present circumstances. The individual expression of charge is a beautiful thing to observe. Helping that charge find both its freedom and its peaceful home in the body is a reward beyond compare, obviously for the client but also for the practitioner.

Nowhere is this dance of charge more intricate than when working with trauma. Here the charge can be massive or barely perceptible. It can take someone apart or bring them back home. Tracking charge in trauma is like playing a game of hide-and-seek—now you see it, now you don't, leading ever deeper into the mystery of human consciousness. Helping a client manage their charge from traumatic situations is a delicate art, similar to dismantling a bomb while the seconds tick away near the end of a movie. It must be done skillfully and carefully, avoiding explosion, while untangling the "wired-up" cycles of negativity.

While a full discussion of trauma and a description of how to work with it goes beyond the scope of this book, I mention it here because *the management of charge figures prominently in the treatment of trauma.* And while simple charging and discharging exercises are helpful for the average individual, one must proceed much more cautiously when working with those suffering from trauma or post–traumatic stress disorder (PTSD).

The discussion that follows will focus primarily on the issue of how to handle *charge* in trauma. And while I have studied with various teachers and writers on the subject, I owe a great debt to my training many years ago with Peter Levine in what was then called Somatic Experiencing. My work with individuals was transformed by what I learned there and has given me an even deeper understanding of charge and how to work with it. Much of what I say on the following pages is adapted from Peter's pioneering work on the subject.

What Makes Something Traumatic?

Our nervous systems are hardwired for self-protection. We shiver when it's cold and sweat when we're hot. We jump at loud sounds and naturally orient our attention to any sudden movements that catch our eye. When we feel threatened, the body floods with charge, giving us both heightened awareness and the energy to take action, all for the purpose of ensuring our survival. Once survival is guaranteed, and the threat is resolved or removed, we can return to a base level of charge that brings us back into balance. (We will explore survival instincts more closely in Chakra One, Chapter 11.)

Trauma occurs when the nervous system is overwhelmed and our self-protective instincts fail to complete their job of self-protection. That's a fancy way of saying that trauma occurs when something awful happens that we are powerless to stop.

Perhaps the situation is so frightening that our innate reactions do not even arise but remain frozen or disabled at the core of the body, described by the phrase "scared stiff." Many people have experienced this, in dreams if not in reality: feeling rooted to the spot, unable to move, or trying to scream but unable to make a sound. The expression "acting like a deer in headlights" illustrates this freezing response. One is unable to think clearly or take effective action. It's not that the charge isn't there—it's that it's locked up.

Sometimes the self-protective instincts do arise, but we face a threat bigger than we can handle. We quickly realize we have to override our natural inclinations to run away or fight someone off, because such actions could make matters worse. This occurs for small children facing a "giant" parent's rage; for anyone facing the threat of a gun or a gang of attackers; or for someone who sees a truck speeding toward them in the wrong lane. In these instances, there is little you can do, so the self-protective instincts that do arise don't get to complete their actions. Yet the intense charge that accompanies them still arises.

Some traumas seem obvious, such as rape, war, physical violence, or sexual abuse. But there are many other instances that can be traumatic, such as surgeries (especially as a child), car accidents, sports injuries, dental procedures, bullying, public humiliation, prolonged immobility, severe illnesses, severe intimidation, verbal abuse, and extreme neglect. Trauma can occur from an intense experience that happens only once, such as a rape or a car accident, or it can occur from less intense experiences that happen repeatedly, such as a child who is emotionally traumatized by constant criticism or rejection. Trauma can also occur from an experience that lasts a long time, such as a young child who has to endure casts on her legs, someone confined by a long-term illness or incarceration, or an extended separation from a parent or loved one, especially at a young age. Trauma can occur from sudden or extreme loss, like the death of a loved one, or loss of one's home or village due to a natural disaster, or even witnessing someone else being hurt. And finally, there can be developmental trauma when a child fails to receive what he needs to adequately complete important stages of childhood development.

The point, however, is not so much in the kinds of things that can *cause* trauma, as it is the nervous system's *response* to the situation. When the nervous system becomes overwhelmed and incapacitated, a person can become traumatized. If someone is able to triumph over their situation, such as by fighting off the attacker, running to safety, or otherwise mobilizing their energy toward resolution, then trauma is less likely to occur.

What Happens to the Charge?

In trauma, the high charge that arises in the body can't be discharged through action. Instead, the charge spins around in a vortex of energy that can impact any aspect of mind, body, emotion, or spirit. The charge is then bound into the tissues, behavior patterns, emotional states, or obsessive thoughts. Peter Levine calls this a *trauma vortex*—a swirling disturbance of energy within the normal stream of experience.

While it may seem counterintuitive, a person may *unconsciously* seek out circumstances similar to the original trauma, such as marrying someone who turns out to be violent or alcoholic like one's dad, having multiple car accidents, or putting oneself into some kind of danger. I say *unconsciously* because who in their right mind would choose to expose themselves to a traumatizing situation? It's as if the soul is still seeking the release that was impossible in the original situation and tries to do that by re-creating a similar pattern. But there's a paradox here. The charge that arises may be seeking release, but instead the similar situation tends to reinforce the defenses, leaving a person even more locked up than before.

If that defense is a freezing response, then almost any situation of high charge—even excitement about something good—could potentially trigger the freezing response. If the defense is fight or flight, you could get triggered into this reaction by an argument with a spouse, a challenge at work, or anything else that naturally brings up your charge. Suddenly the whole body is ready to run away or punch someone out. When these responses happen, they often seem out of the person's control, as if we are riding in a car that someone else is driving.

Three Pathways of Charge

Stephen Porges, originator of the Polyvagal Theory of Emotion,[2] suggests that there are three basic neural pathways that can be activated when a person feels threatened. These channels of response occur through various branches of the vagus nerve, a major cranial nerve that activates parts of the brain, as well as influencing the heart, lungs, digestive system, and muscular expression. The three branches produce three different reactions to trauma or a later triggering of traumatic memory.

1. *Shutdown*

    The oldest pathway, evolutionarily speaking, creates a physiological "shutdown." In the animal world, it can be an attempt to "play dead" to keep from being seen or attacked. This is the *freeze response*. We might lose our capacity to think, feel, or take action. We could be rooted to the spot, unable to step forward or move our limbs. Sometimes during surgeries, car accidents, or extreme trauma, individuals experience floating above their body, completely dissociated from what's happening.

    This shutdown is a biological mechanism that lessens the impact of pain and terror by numbing the body. But it's not something we can control. It happens of its own accord when this aspect of the vagus nerve is aroused. The feeling of being out of control can create shame or even greater fear in a person. This explains why people often look back at a trauma and wonder why they didn't do more to stop it. They might feel angry with themselves over this failure to act, without realizing this is a biological response that takes over when necessary.

In PTSD, the shutdown mechanism may occur in future instances when no actual trauma is taking place. This happens when someone has flashbacks from war trauma or "checks out" while having sex. Because the freeze response halts things like digestion or deep breathing, it can sometimes create lifelong physiological problems, including pain and blocked energy.

I remember an embarrassing evening back in my twenties, when I was playing electric piano in an all-women's rock band. When it came time for my solo, the anxiety of the moment shot me into an altered state. I couldn't remember what song we were playing, what key it was in, or what I was supposed to be doing. I could barely make my fingers move. The audience seemed distant and faraway, as if in a dream. I couldn't remember my band members' names. I felt such shame about it I didn't want to face my bandmates. Shortly after, I stopped playing music publicly and made it just a hobby. I now know I had gone into a freeze response, triggered by the high charge of the situation, even though no danger was actually present.

2. *Fight or Flight*

The next pathway in the polyvagal theory prepares the body for fight or flight. Here the stress hormones flood the bloodstream, the heart races, and the muscles are readied for action. The important point here is that the charge floods the body in preparation for fight or flight, but when it can't be "spent" in activity, it keeps the body in a perpetual state of defensive readiness—a state highly stressful for the body. A person may even find themselves "looking for a fight" or scanning for danger.

When the body gets locked into this state, the high charge gets locked in as well, but more consciously seeks to be released. A person might try to discharge through obsessive workout routines, running, or gambling. Because the body experiences fear, even when no present threat exists, the mind will look outward for something to justify that fear. I often tell my clients, "Just because you feel fear in your body doesn't mean there's anything to be afraid of." But the inner state speaks louder than my words.

3. *Social Connection*

The third and more recent evolutionary response is to seek social connection. This part of the vagus nerve activates the voice, middle ear, and facial muscles. Shelley Taylor's theory that men go to "fight or flight" while women are more likely to "tend and befriend" may be reflecting this third path to social connection. (However, both women and men are subject to any of these polyvagal responses.)

When social cues signify safety, such as a mother comforting her child, the more primitive responses are inhibited, and social connection can take place. But the converse can also be true: When one is experiencing shutdown or caught in a state of fight or flight, these states can hijack the ability to connect socially. When you're triggered, it's difficult to be soft, open, and intimate. (We'll look more deeply at charge patterns in relationship in Chapter 24.)

Working with Charge in Trauma

To heal trauma, one has to discharge, albeit carefully. The safest way to proceed is to discharge in small, discrete packets, similar to letting the steam off a pressure cooker before the lid is opened. It's essential to know how to track a person's charge to do this effectively. Working with trauma takes considerable training, and this is but a brief presentation, but here are some guidelines.

Establish Safety

When I work with a client on issues of trauma, I start with establishing a sense of safety by taking time to create connection and rapport. I do this through listening deeply and reflecting back what I hear with genuine interest and compassion.

I then ask the client to think of a time in her life where she felt safe, powerful, loved, peaceful, happy, or connected. If she says, "When I'm walking on the beach with my dog," or "Visiting my grandmother in the country," then I ask her to immerse herself in this imagined scene and explore what it feels like as she does so. I look carefully to see if this memory is effective. Do I notice that she's relaxing? Do I see her breath deepen, her body becoming quieter? Do I feel her become more present? Does she seem more at ease? If so, I know I have found a "resource" I can bring her back to, a way to calm her nervous system.

If the image doesn't work to bring this relaxation, I look for something else to use, until I find something that works. If someone can't think of such a time—perhaps they have no memory at all of feeling safe or loved—then I ask them to invent one. They could imagine being protected by a dragon, floating peacefully on a cloud, or living on the moon. It doesn't have to be realistic; it just has to create a feeling of relaxation, safety, peace, or well-being.

Facilitate Small Discharges

Next I begin small discharges of whatever is present before even talking about the trauma. Often in workshops, a person's charge goes sky-high just because they have volunteered to work in front of the group. I don't want to go into a trauma memory with all that charge present. So I might have them push into my hands, kick their feet, run in place, or make some soft sounds, until I see their charge come back down to a manageable level.

Then I proceed slowly, starting at the far outskirts of the trauma. If it was a car accident that happened coming home from work, I might start with what was going on that morning before the person left the house. Maybe they were having an argument with their spouse and the charge of that memory arises as they talk about it. I then discharge that small amount of charge until things are neutral again and the person is relaxed and present.

Once a person returns to equilibrium, I can take a step closer to the trauma but still remain on the outskirts. "How was your mood at work the day of the accident? How did you feel as you walked into the parking lot at the end of the day?" Once again, I discharge any activation that I see, never allowing the person to get too highly charged, never straying too far from equilibrium. This keeps the charge manageable at all times and allows the client to feel empowered.

As the story unfolds slowly toward the point of trauma, the packets of charge may become more intense. Still, I release them in small steps, often slowing the client down with a statement like, "Let's stop right there and just breathe for a moment. What do you notice in your body?" Once the charge has been acknowledged, the client then has the option to release another small piece of it.

Restore Instinctual Responses

Because charge activates various parts of the body for some kind of action, I might ask that part of the body what it wants to do. For instance, if a person notices her hands are becoming shaky, I might ask her what the hands want to do. Maybe they want to push something away or pull someone close. If possible, I give the hands something to push into or to pull on—often my own hands, giving slight resistance. Again, I wait for the return to equilibrium, pausing in each state of relaxation before going on.

Savor the Quiet Moments

I want to anchor the states of equilibrium between the small discharges. I might say, "I see your breath becoming more relaxed now, your shoulders dropping down. Let's pause here and really feel that sense of relaxation." There's no hurry to move forward.

It's more important to allow the pleasurable sensations to sink in, to begin to rewire the brain's habit of fear and activation and create a new experience of calm in the nervous system. It is also possible to create this by revisiting the positive memory to anchor this relaxation.

Unravel the Trauma

At the heart of a traumatic memory, there is a potent vortex of charge. Because it hasn't yet been released, it tends to go around and around in an unproductive cycle, an energetic vortex that exists outside the stream of time. Present time can proceed all around us, but when we're caught in a trauma vortex, we may be wrapped up in something that happened when we were five years old as if it were yesterday.

It may take several sessions of releasing discrete packets of charge before a client is neutralized enough to be able to walk through the center of a trauma vortex. I never hurry to get to this place, but let it unfold naturally, constantly tracking the charge to make sure it stays near the comfort zone. It might happen in that session, or it might be weeks away.

Unraveling the trauma may involve making sound, moving the body, shaking, pushing, stomping, or being protected, such as wrapping up in a blanket. It is not for me, as a practitioner, to say what is right for that person's release but instead to follow the body's natural inclinations and allow them to occur in a manner slow and safe enough to be tolerated without the person becoming overcharged.

Renegotiate the Trauma

Once a trauma is sufficiently discharged, the healing process can proceed in a new direction. Instead of moving *toward* the trauma, releasing packets of discharge along the way, the person can now re-create a more positive experience and move away from the trauma. Sometimes I take a person through an alternate experience of growing up, with statements such as, "Imagine now that you have this protection as a three-year-old. What would feel different in your three-year-old body?" Then I take it forward in time.

"Now imagine if you had that protection at three, what it would have felt like to go to kindergarten at five years old . . . to be in the third grade . . . to enter middle school . . . high school . . . go off to college . . . get married?"

Of course, this proceeds slowly, allowing the person to "install" the new program of safety, power, love, protection, or self-reliance at each stage. I often say, "Soak your cells in that experience," to make sure the fantasy gets lodged in the body. The important point is not whether it actually happened but to install the *feeling* that would have occurred, had the positive scenario taken place.

Until the trauma is discharged, however, this alternate reality may be impossible to imagine. It simply won't stick, as the charge is holding the old pattern in place. It's after the grief or the terror has been released that the components of memory can be rearranged.

Can You Do This for Yourself?

Years ago, I had a car accident, in which I broke two ribs and punctured a lung. Needless to say, I was somewhat traumatized, and my ribs were so sore, the slightest movement of my torso would cause searing pain. After about a month of healing, I woke up in the middle of the night and knew I needed to thrash about. By then my body was strong enough to twist and turn at least a little. I could release sounds and small movements, and facilitate a discharge. Because I was trained in trauma, I knew exactly what I was doing. I knew to follow the impulses of my body and to not do it all at once.

I had the thought at the time that most people would not know what to do with that impulse. Most likely they would repress their instincts toward discharge, or they might feel shame about shaking or making strange sounds in the middle of the night!

In general, however, it is difficult to heal one's own trauma without outside assistance from a trained therapist. That's because we may be unable to handle the intense triggers to our charge, or we're unable to interrupt the freezing response or the fight/flight activation.

If a traumatic memory should surface unexpectedly, it helps to have a little knowledge about how to handle it. Befriend the charge and notice what it wants to do. Discharge it in small, manageable packets, and be patient enough to go slowly, moving toward healing over time. As you return to a more regulated state, anchor the feeling of calm and safety in your body.

Managing the Comfort Zone

While working with trauma is a delicate art, the main point I want to make is that there is often a tremendous amount of charge that, when reawakened, can re-create the original feelings of helplessness, freezing, or activation. It is essential to avoid leading a client into repeated experiences of helplessness by going straight into the trauma and expecting them to release it all at once. It is far better to assist them in managing their charge in small enough packets that they are not pushed out of their comfort zone and can maintain safety and develop self-mastery. Because many therapists and bodyworkers may stumble onto trauma unexpectedly, without any training in how to deal with it, remembering the simple rule to "proceed slowly and safely" can be a gentle guide.

part iii

CHARGE
and the
CHAKRAS

chapter 10

ARCHITECTURE
of the
SOUL

IIIIIIIIIIIIIIIIIIIIIIIIIIIIIIIIIIIIIIIIIIIII

Charge and the Chakra System

*Allow a deep sense of awe to fill your awareness as you
perceive the gravity and beauty of your soul's awakening.*

JAMES O'DEA

At the sacred center of each one of us, spin seven wheels of
vital energy, called *chakras*. Aligned vertically along the energetic
core of the body, the chakra system is an organizational structure
for how the soul handles its life force. I call it the *architecture of
the soul*. Each chakra is a chamber in the temple of your body that
handles a particular kind of energy, much like the different rooms
in your home handle distinct energies. If we are going to work
with charge and the energy body, we need to understand its basic
architecture.

The chakras manage charge in forms that span the full spectrum of human experience: from your primal instincts, to your
emotions, actions, relationships, communication, and vision,
on to your highest consciousness. I've written extensively about

chakra philosophy and psychology in my other books.** Here we'll look specifically at how the chakras handle charge, along with exercises for charging and discharging, and ultimately balancing. If you are new to the chakras, this chapter serves as a primer. If you are already familiar with chakra theory, you may want to skip to Chapters 11–17, focusing on each chakra in turn, where you will likely gain new material.

The Chakras as a System of Energy

The word *chakra* comes from Sanskrit, the ancient language of India, and literally means *wheel* or *disk*. Though this was not a metaphor known to the ancients, these wheels are like the old-fashioned floppy disks we once used in our computers. Each chakra handles a different set of programs—such as our relationship program, our language program, or the images or feelings stored in memory.

Chakras exist at the meeting point of mind and body, in what is called the subtle body, yet they have a location in the physical body, as seen in Figure 7. As we know from Chapter 2, *energy is the interface between consciousness and the physical body.* Even though chakras are not physical, like an organ or bone, the chakras do influence your experience of the physical body. Butterflies in your stomach, a frog in your throat, or an ache in your back can be attributed to the influence of the chakras in those areas.

** For a quick introduction to the chakras, see *Chakras: Seven Keys to Awakening and Healing the Energy Body* (London: Hay House, 2016). For more about basic chakra philosophy, see *Wheels of Life: A User's Guide to the Chakra System* (St. Paul, MN: Llewellyn Publications, 1987). For more about chakra psychology, see *Eastern Body, Western Mind: Psychology and the Chakra System as a Path to the Self* (Berkeley, CA: Celestial Arts, 2004). For more about chakras and yoga, see *Anodea Judith's Chakra Yoga* (St. Paul, MN: Llewellyn Publications, 2016).

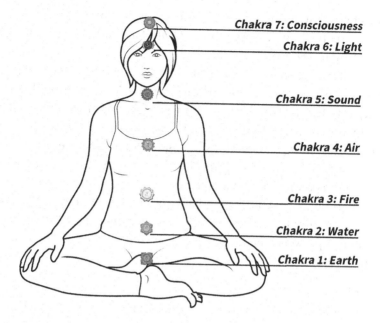

Chakra 7: Consciousness

Chakra 6: Light

Chakra 5: Sound

Chakra 4: Air

Chakra 3: Fire

Chakra 2: Water

Chakra 1: Earth

Figure 7 Chakra Elements

My working definition of a chakra is this:

A chakra is an organizational center for the reception, assimilation, storage, and expression of life force energy, or charge.

Each chakra manages a different kind of energy and is associated with a particular element. In fact, the elements are the simplest way to understand the function of each chakra, as these elements exist both within us and around us (Figure 7). Earth, at the bottom, is solid. That's our foundation. Water is fluid and gets energy moving. Fire turns energy into power; breath is expansive; sound is a vibration, light an even higher vibration, and consciousness, a limitless nonmaterial essence.

The chakras are primary gateways for both charging and discharging and act as portals between the inner and outer worlds. But as receivers and senders of energy, the chakras are not wide-open portals that take everything in or let everything out. Instead, they are intelligent patterns in the body/mind system that filter and check energy as it enters and leaves the body, much like a doorman checks who comes in and out of a building. They do this according to their programming.

Chakras receive energy from the outer world, then "digest" that energy and incorporate it into the physical, emotional, energetic, intellectual, or spiritual bodies. You might say they "step energy down" from the universal to the particular, the way a solar panel takes energy from the sun and turns it into electricity for your home. Chakras can then either store that energy for future use (such as a memory or a feeling), or they discharge it through action and expression. To be healthy, each chakra needs to be able to perform all four of these functions—*reception, assimilation, storage, and expression*—at its particular level of being. Let's look at each of these in more detail.

Reception

As a chakra receives energy, it filters what comes in. The throat chakra, which processes communication, receives the words someone is saying but may selectively listen, hearing only what we want to hear. In the second chakra, we receive sensate experience but sort out what feels good versus what feels bad. In the crown chakra, we might filter information as it comes in, discarding that which doesn't go with our worldview.

Obviously, we need to be able to open and receive through our chakras in order to remain healthy and energized. If we filter too much, we lose our capacity to receive fully. If we don't filter enough, we get overloaded with more input than we can process or assimilate.

Assimilation

Chakras are also the *assimilators* of energy into the core. They process our experience, thoughts, beliefs, and emotions, much as our digestive system assimilates our food and turns it into nutrients and calories. If we can't incorporate what we receive, it slows down the chakra's energy, like a computer chewing on a big file or a belly trying to digest a Thanksgiving dinner. But sometimes we don't have the capacity to integrate something. This can happen when someone is speaking to you in a foreign language, or it can happen to a child who can't assimilate the anger of his parents or learn lessons beyond his stage of development.

If you eat food, are you able to digest that food and make good use of it? If someone gives you love or support, are you able to take that in and remember later that you are loved? If you are learning a new subject, are you able to understand and integrate what you are learning? Have you ever had a conversation with someone who seemed to be listening but afterward behaved as if they hadn't heard a word you said? Even if you receive and express charge through your chakras, the ability to *keep that charge* and turn it into something valuable depends on your ability to assimilate and store the energy.

Storage

Just as calories can be stored as fat, chakras can *store* energy in the form of body structure, emotions, habits, and memory. You could say that chakras store the energies and programming of our complexes, running them again and again, the way a computer stores programs on the hard drive. If the drive is too full, we don't have room to store anything more and are stuck running old programs. And if our storage capacity is too small, like a tiny closet with no shelves or a hard drive with too little memory, then we have no place to put anything.

Expression

And finally, chakras *express* energy. We tell somebody what we're feeling, or we take action after planning our strategy. If we can't express energy through a chakra, we can't discharge, and that in turn limits what we can take in.

In this complicated sorting process, the chakras build up defenses between the inner and outer worlds. These defenses were created to keep external energy out and vital energy in. If we think what's inside us is not okay, such as holding the belief that we're stupid or not trusting our emotions, then the chakras inhibit what is expressed or discharged and keep that energy in.

If you were carrying strong emotion at a time when it was either unsafe or inappropriate to let that emotion out, you would defend against the *discharge* of that emotion. We all do this in situations where getting angry or having a crying jag isn't a good idea. But if you grew up in an environment where it *never* felt safe to express emotion, this habit would also get hardwired into the body. It might be through a holding pattern lodged in the second chakra, which handles emotion, or perhaps a pattern that holds back in the throat chakra, the area of self-expression, or perhaps makes you afraid to take action, the realm of the third chakra.

So we can see that the chakras are very busy handling energy, through receiving, sorting, integrating, storing, and expressing charge. And since that energy can take many forms, both positive and negative, or more often mixtures of both, the seven chakras form some pretty complex patterns in the architecture of each person's soul. Working with the chakras requires a deep understanding of the role each center plays in handling charge.

Chakras as Storage Pouches

We have stated how the body is a storage battery for charge. Chakras can store our experiences, memories, habits, and beliefs—all of which have a certain amount of charge. Memories that have strong charge—such as a traumatic memory—consequently store more charge in various parts of the body. This can work positively or negatively. Storing the energy of someone's love can comfort you in times of despair, or you can store up anger that erupts suddenly when you don't want it to.

If you think of the vertical core of the body as a great big tube in which energy travels up and down and you want to store energy in any part of that tube, you would need to create a place to put it. Just as an elevator goes up and down between floors but doesn't really store energy (it just lets people on and off at each floor), the core handles the transportation of charge up and down the chakra system, between heaven and earth, mind and body, spirit and matter. But the core is just a conduit for charge—it doesn't store it, except through the chakras. Like a straw, the energy can rise and fall, but unless you create some kind of "storage pouch" along the way, there is no mechanism for keeping energy partway up or down.

So you can think of the chakras as energetic storage pouches along the core of the body, where you find not only gates that defend what passes through but an energetic "space" to store what is assimilated, so that it can become part of the basic body structure, memory, or behaviors. (see Figure 8 below). That space isn't a literal space—you couldn't dissect the body and find it—but it is an energetic sense of openness and expansion.

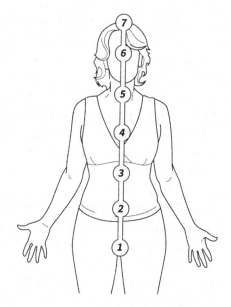

Figure 8 Chakras as Storage Pouches for Charge

Excessive and Deficient Chakras

Chakras can heighten or diminish charge, much like the capacitors and resistors of electronic equipment. If the habit is to not feel your emotions or your sexuality, the second chakra will constrict to minimize energy at that level. This will create resistance and slow down everything flowing through the second chakra, maybe even resulting in lower back pain. If the habit is to live in your head, trying to figure things out intellectually, you will "rev up" your higher chakras when faced with a problem and pull energy out of your lower chakras. Then perhaps the throat chakra constricts to keep energy in the storage pouch of the head from moving down into the body.

A chakra's ability to properly assimilate energy depends on a balanced level of charging and discharging. If a chakra is receiving more energy than it can discharge, then it would become "excessively" charged. If your throat chakra were overcharged, for example, you would be excessively focused on talking, or maybe the energy would be blocked up in your neck and shoulders. There is a lot of "energy" there, but it's stagnant. In an excessive chakra, there is too much packed inside for it to flow smoothly.

A deficient chakra, by contrast, starts to close down, making a smaller "storage pouch," or crimping the tube that runs from heaven to earth, blocking the passage up and down. Even when there's a possibility of taking energy in, it's not able to do so—there's simply not enough room to store it. It's like offering a truckload of furniture to a person living in a small apartment. They literally have no way to receive it.

Of course, it's not always so cut-and-dried. Some chakras have characteristics of both excess and deficiency at the same time in different aspects of that chakra. For instance, the second chakra, which is said to handle both emotions and sexuality, could show a pattern of someone who is highly sexual and not very emotional, or the reverse, highly emotional and not very sexual. This is simply another pattern of the person's attempt to balance their charge within that chakra.

Both excess and deficiency in the chakras are a result of a defensive strategy that modulates the energy coming in and out. Excess results from a *compensating* strategy—meaning we compensate for something we didn't get enough of, like love or feeling powerful, overdoing our focus on that issue. A deficient chakra results from an *avoidant* strategy. We want to avoid feeling our emotions, taking action, or dealing with an issue.

So you see, there are many aspects to understanding the chakras as mediators of energy, with patterns that differ from person to person. Much like the human face, where the eyes are always above the nose, there are universal aspects to the chakra system, but each person has a personal expression that is unique.

What follows is a more detailed look at the various ways that each chakra handles charge.

THE CHAKRA SYSTEM

CHAKRA	LOCATION	CENTRAL ISSUE	GOALS	RIGHTS	DEVELOPMENT STAGE
7	Top of head, cerebral cortex	Awareness	Wisdom, knowledge, consciousness, spiritual connection	To know	Throughout life
6	Brow	Intuition, Imagination	Psychic perception, accurate interpretation, imagination, seeing	To see	Adolescence
5	Throat	Communication	Clear communication, creativity, resonance	To speak and be heard	7 to 12 years
4	Heart	Love, Relationships	Balance, compassion, self-acceptance, good relationships	To love and be loved	4 to 7 years
3	Solar plexus	Power, Will	Vitality, spontaneity, strength of will, purpose, self-esteem	To act	18 months to 4 years
2	Abdomen, genitals, lower back, hips	Sexuality, Emotions	Fluidity, pleasure, healthy sexuality, feeling function	To feel, to want	6 months to 2 years
1	Base of spine, coccygeal plexus	Survival	Stability, grounding, physical health, prosperity, trust	To be here, to have	Womb to 12 months

DENTITY	DEMON	EXCESSIVE CHARACTERISTICS	DEFICIENT CHARACTERISTICS	ELEMENT
Universal Self-nowledge)	Attachment	Overly intellectual, spiritual addiction, confusion, dissociated body	Learning difficulties, spiritual skepticism, limited beliefs, materialism, apathy	Conscious Thought
rchetypal elf-eflection)	Illusion	Headaches, nightmares, hallucinations, delusions, difficulty concentrating	Poor memory, poor vision, cannot see patterns, denial	Light
reative elf-pression)	Lies	Excessive talking, inability to listen, overextended, stuttering	Fear of speaking, poor rhythm, aphasia	Sound
cial (Self-ceptance)	Grief	Codependency, poor boundaries, possessive, jealous, narcissistic	Shy, lonely, isolated, lack of empathy, bitter, critical	Air
o (Self-fintion)	Shame	Dominating, blaming, aggressive, scattered, constantly active	Weak will, poor self-esteem, passive, sluggish, fearful	Fire
otional lf-tification)	Guilt	Overly emotional, poor boundaries, sex addiction, obsessive attachments	Frigidity, impotence, rigidity, emotional numbness, fear of pleasure	Water
sical lf-servation)	Fear	Heaviness, sluggish, monotony, obesity, hoarding, materialism	Frequent fear, lack of discipline, restless, underweight, spacey	Earth

chapter 11

CHAKRA
One

||||||||||||||||||||||||||||

Fight, Flight, Freeze, or Fold

Human existence rests upon the fact of embodiment.

STANLEY KELEMAN

The first chakra corresponds to the element *earth* and represents the energy of your basic survival instincts. You are born
with these instincts, hardwired into your nervous system. Without them, a newborn would not know how to suckle, the mother
wouldn't know how to care for her child, and the human species
would never have survived. Yet these instincts are by nature primitive: they arise very quickly and run their programs constantly,
mostly below the radar of our awareness.

When something triggers your survival instincts, it's almost
always accompanied by strong charge. That charge has a distinct
purpose in the first chakra: *to make sure the body continues to survive.* It might be the instinct to hunt for food when you're hungry,
to sleep when you're tired, to fight off a predator, or to run away
from danger. All these actions require a tremendous amount of
charge and will literally steal that charge from other parts of the
body, mind, or chakra system when necessary.

In other words, when someone pulls a gun on you and you're running for your life, you don't think about the book you're reading, about how you look, or whether your taxes are paid. Your survival needs take over and all systems rally toward whatever it takes to become safe again.

In crisis, energy is pulled away from your intellect, your digestion, and anything else that might interfere with having enough energy to save your life. Once the danger has passed, the charge returns back to these other levels of the body-mind complex. But if the danger is persistent or ever-present, the charge can become permanently hijacked by the survival instincts. That leaves us in a state of hypervigilance and hair-trigger readiness to respond to any potential danger.

Fight or Flight

Imagine you wake up in the night to a loud noise downstairs in your house. Suspecting it might be a burglar, your body will immediately tense up and flood with charge—regardless of whether the threat is real or imagined. If it turns out it was nothing but the cat knocking over a plant or just a bad dream, your charge would eventually settle back down. Depending on how much you were aroused, the dissipation of charge might take a little while before you completely calm down and get back to sleep.

If, heaven forbid, you realized it really was an intruder, you would then be flooded with even more charge for the purpose of action. You would be compelled to grab something to defend yourself or climb out the window to run away. The charge would intensify your experience, commanding all your consciousness toward staying alive until you felt safe again. If you then "spend" your charge appropriately, fighting the intruder or running away, your charge would eventually return to its baseline level, having been discharged in action.

So we have two patterns here: charge that returns to baseline when it is no longer needed, and charge that returns to baseline because it has been spent or discharged. Either one of these scenarios is natural. The activation of charge is not permanent and generally doesn't tend to cause further problems.

If you examine the basic action of fight or flight, you can see that fighting requires *increasing one's charge* in order to deal with a threat while flight is an attempt to *avoid a threat,* or get away from it before it causes harm. In order to do either one—to fight or to flee—the legs flood with charge. But running away can also take the form of *escaping the experience* of the body, perhaps fleeing up into the head or into compulsive activities or numbing behaviors. That can be another kind of flight, one that pulls energy away from the body and its immediate experience. This kind of flight binds energy away from the first chakra and keeps it depleted.

The Freeze Response

What happens when you can't fight and there's nowhere to run? The charge becomes frozen, often in the legs, but it can also freeze the arms, chest, belly, the emotions, or the ability to think clearly.

Unfortunately, when children are getting yelled at or abused, or when adults are in situations of helplessness, like being held at gunpoint, neither fighting nor fleeing is possible. There may be no way to fight off a parent who is bigger than you or to resist someone holding a gun. You can't fight something beyond your control, like a car accident that takes place in a few split seconds, but neither can you run away. Then you are not able to "spend" your charge in either fight or flight, nor are you able to relax because the danger passes. Yet the charge still arises biologically as a hard-wired response, beyond your conscious control. What happens to all that charge when it can't be spent?

Well, did your computer ever suddenly "freeze" in the midst of writing a document or watching a movie? Do you remember that annoying feeling of having to reboot, sometimes losing valuable information?

In a similar way, the high arousal of charge can "freeze" and immobilize your ability to receive, assimilate, or express energy effectively. This could impact more than just the first chakra's fight or flight. It might create an inability to feel anything (second chakra), it might freeze your impulse toward action (third chakra), or inhibit your breathing (fourth chakra) or undermine your ability to speak up (fifth chakra), or even block your capacity to see or think clearly (sixth and seventh chakras). Any of the chakras and their corresponding levels of response can get frozen when the charge can't be expressed or spent, depending on what may have gotten activated at the time.

In an ideal situation, a person eventually "thaws out" from that frozenness and returns to normal, shaking off the excess charge through movement, sound, or activity. But too often even that is impossible. Sometimes people are exposed to repeated violence, and they can't discharge between the beatings. Sometimes, there is no one to offer supportive guidance for a discharge of emotion or action. Then the charge remains frozen until it is eventually bound into the body somewhere, relegated to the unconscious and hidden from awareness.

This is the case with posttraumatic stress disorder (PTSD), which we discussed in the section on trauma (Chapter 9). For now, let's consider freezing as a kind of blockage that is *rooted in* (but not limited to) the base chakra's survival programming, as a third component of the fight-or-flight syndrome. This freezing often makes healthy programming unavailable—just like when your computer freezes, your documents and operating system become inaccessible. Sure, we can reboot, but if the program bug isn't addressed, it will happen repeatedly, undermining general functionality.

The fight-or-flight response creates an excessive state of energy in the first chakra.

The Fold Response

Now let's see what happens when a person's energy freezes and an unfortunate scenario actually does take place. A person may *collapse* under the strain and disconnect from their charge entirely. This gives a fourth possibility: fight, flight, freeze, or *fold*. Folding is a kind of resignation, self-abandonment, or collapse. It looks like the charge disappears from the body, leaving a person feeling cold, empty, vacant, or depleted. It's very similar to blowing a fuse in your home when a circuit becomes overloaded—the circuit breaker simply shuts off the current, and the lights go out. Alternatively, such a collapse might be a person's way of trying to minimize the impact of the negative experience, much the way we look away when the doctor is giving us a shot with a needle. When the body can't run away, often the energy takes flight instead.

A fold response may appear as if there is little or no charge at all, yet the charge is still locked in the body somewhere, just dissociated from consciousness. The body may exhibit a collapsed or slumped posture, muscles that do not hold their tone, or you may see emotional flatness or a vacant, disconnected feeling of self. Then the survival instincts remain inactivated, even when needed. Such a person may have difficulty setting boundaries, being assertive, manifesting what they need to survive, or even noticing the needs of their body, needs as basic as eating and sleeping.

The fold response creates a deficient state in the first chakra.

Stress Hormones and Body Chemistry

What's happening physiologically in the body when survival is threatened?

When danger threatens, two systems are activated simultaneously: the *sympathetic nervous system* through the pathway of the nerves and the *adrenal cortical system* through the release of chemicals into the bloodstream. The sympathetic nervous system creates a state of tension and alertness, preparing the body for action. Your muscles tighten, your eyes widen, and your palms get sweaty. The cortical system releases epinephrine (adrenaline) and norepinephrine, (noradrenaline). These chemicals (along with estrogen, testosterone, cortisol, and some 30 other chemicals) increase heart rate and blood pressure, so that more energy gets to the cells faster for the action required.

Additionally, anything peripheral, such as digestion or immune functions, will shut down, so as not to usurp energy needed for defense. The pupils dilate in order to take in more light, sugars are released from the liver for energy, and smooth muscles relax, allowing greater capacity for the lungs to take in more oxygen.

This is all designed to generate energy for fight or flight. Whew! For an instantaneous reflex, that's quite a lot going on! And when this process is either thwarted or activated repeatedly, it creates permanent patterns, lodged into the whole body-mind complex. We feel like we're constantly in a survival state of consciousness, hypervigilant, ready to run at any moment, unable to relax. This stress can wear down the organs, exhaust the adrenals, contribute to heart disease, imbalance blood sugar levels, and cause general wear and tear on the body. Far too many people live in this state.

Freezing the Roots

The legs are the roots of the spine. They connect the root chakra to the ground, a few feet below. We can only be fully grounded when the legs are able to make dynamic contact with the ground, moving the charge both up from the earth and down to the earth.

When survival energies are aroused, it not only sends energy up the spine but also downward, to activate the legs, so they can run or kick if necessary. If the energy becomes frozen, the channels of the legs may also freeze, and the legs can no longer appropriately carry the charge between the base of the spine and the earth. The first chakra becomes essentially blocked. It can neither receive nor discharge.

This makes it difficult, if not impossible, to really ground yourself. Grounding is the ability to make dynamic contact with the earth and create solidity and stability in your life. Without grounding, our ability to handle charge is limited, just as we always have a grounding circuit on a power tool that handles more voltage.

Lack of grounding effects our survival functioning. Our instincts askew, we may find ourselves later in life having a difficult time making a living or keeping our physical health balanced. In addition, eating disorders may arise, since eating is basically a survival instinct. We might become excessively focused on survival issues, eating too much, or avoid the feeling of solidity in the body altogether and eat too little. (However, eating disorders are too complex to be relegated to a single chakra.)

If we choose compensating strategies for this blockage (excessive first chakra), then we tend to hyperfocus on aspects related to the earth plane: we hang on to material goods, even creating clutter; we may eat too much and gain weight, creating a more substantial body; or we may become overly focused on money and finance, hoarding or lavishing our wealth.

If we instead choose the fleeing or leaving response (deficient first chakra), then we tend to ignore issues related to the earth plane. We might make a lighter body, avoid eating, deal poorly with finances, have difficulty manifesting, or be so flighty we never stay long in one place.

Remember, excessive chakras carry too much charge and are a result of compensation for a wound or difficulty, while deficient chakras are an avoidant response to the energies of a particular chakra.

What to Do?

To balance the first chakra's ability to appropriately charge, assimilate, store, and discharge, the leg channels need to be opened. Think of the legs as the two prongs of a plug that we must plug into the circuit of the earth plane. Because matter is densely stored energy, when we push down against what is solid, we draw up energy.

More appropriate to the first chakra's Sanskrit name, *Muladhara*, which means "root support," you can think of the legs as the roots of the first chakra. Roots bring energy *up* from the earth and simultaneously push energy *down* into the earth. When roots draw energy from the earth into the plant, it represents the feminine aspect of nourishment, drawing water and nutrients up from the soil. The aspect of pushing roots down into the earth represents the masculine aspect of penetration. Whatever our gender, we need to develop both aspects of our roots.

If these channels are not open and flowing, receiving and expressing earth energy can be compromised. Without this connection, we simply don't feel grounded, safe, or relaxed. Our consciousness remains at a primitive and instinctual survival level.

We develop our ground by opening the channels in the legs, so that they can carry charge to and from the earth.

Exercise:

Opening the Leg Channels

1. Begin by standing with your feet parallel, shoulder width apart. After looking down and making sure your feet are wide enough apart (most people make too narrow a base), press your heels out a little wider than your toes, becoming a bit pigeon-toed.

2. Soften your knees, slightly bending out over the second toe, so that you can look down and spot your big toenail just inside your kneecap.

3. Now that your placement is correct press *down and out* with your feet, as if you were trying to push apart the floorboards or stretch the carpet. Feel how the resistance of your feet allows your body to become firmly grounded through your legs.

   This is your basic grounding stance. Now we are going to increase the charge in your legs.

4. As you inhale, slowly bend your knees farther, keeping your shoulders directly over your hips. No need to take your hips as low as your knees; just bending a few inches will suffice. Imagine pulling earth energy *up* your legs, into your first chakra.

5. As you exhale, slowly push *through* the core of each leg as you imagine pushing roots into the earth. Your legs will naturally extend and straighten, but make sure to avoid straightening them all the way or locking your knees, as that will shut off the charge you are trying to build. Straighten your knees about 90 percent of the way, but not 100 percent.

6. Repeat steps four and five *slowly,* coordinating with your inhalation and exhalation (inhale as you bend, exhale as you straighten). Continue to press down and out with your feet slightly pigeon-toed.

7. If you are doing this correctly, you will begin to feel a subtle trembling in your legs. That's exactly what is meant to happen. Allow that trembling to take place—surrender to it. As you continue the exercise, the trembling will increase. Find out just how much bending and straightening, or just what speed increases that trembling and let it happen. This is a sign that new charge is coming into the legs.

8. If you are comfortable keeping that charge or allowing it into the body proper, then go ahead and do so. If you feel uncomfortable or anxious from too much charge, then simply discharge by stomping your feet or running in place.

Excess and Deficiency

A person with an excessive first chakra tends to have too much earth energy, which makes the energy heavy and hard to ignite. The body puts on weight; there is attraction or even addiction to eating, hoarding, or other forms of materiality. As the body becomes heavy, charge is bound into the tissues. It then becomes difficult to activate that charge, to burn up the fat it is stored in and get the body moving. Excessive first chakras result in fixed, stubborn behavior that fears change.

By contrast, a deficient first chakra exhibits a lack of earth energy: poor grounding, a thin body, hypervigilance, and an inability to focus or be still. The wiry, thin body wants to keep moving and lacks a sense of embodied safety. With a deficient first chakra, a person often compensates by excessive upper chakras, living in their heads, escaping through spirituality, or avoidance of embodiment in general.

chapter 12

CHAKRA
Two

||||||||||||||||||||||||||||

Feeling Your Way through Sensations, Emotions, and Sexuality

The life of the body is feeling: feeling alive, vibrant, good, excited, angry, sad, joyous, and finally contented.

ALEXANDER LOWEN

Once we have facilitated charge coming *into* the body, through the legs, we now want to help it flow *through* the body. Facilitating the fluid movement of energy is a primary task of the second chakra, located in the abdominal area, including the hips, lower back, pelvis, and genitals. Here we find our emotional charge, our erotic charge, and our drive toward pleasure and freedom.

Where the first chakra is oriented to survival—keeping the body alive—the second chakra's drive is toward pleasure—feeling good.

It makes sense. Once survival is taken care of and the workday is done, most people want to relax or have fun. Taking this a step further, pain generally makes the body contract, freezing the charge, while pleasure invites us to expand, which melts the frozen charge into a flowing river of energy. We move from solid to liquid by melting. In order to melt, we need to feel safe, with a secure sense of ground below us.

This chakra relates to the element water, and its name, *Svadhisthana,* means "one's own place." Feelings and emotions that stir in the watery depths of this chakra are felt from within our body—in our own place. We occupy this place by feeling the charge that flows there, whether it's emotional charge, erotic charge, or simply energy passing through on its way up the spine. We get knocked out of our own place by being told, "You have no right to feel that way," or by having to distort or repress our emotions. Then we no longer trust the important information coming to us through this chakra. We get out of touch with our own place.

In this chapter, we'll examine the way charge relates to *sensations, emotions,* and *sexuality.* When these aspects of life are in balance, there is a natural flow of charge through the second chakra, with an overall balance between charging and discharging. Each of these aspects plays an important role in our well-being.

Sensation

Lose your mind and come to your senses.

FRITZ PERLS

Your body is immersed in a sea of sensation. Temperature, color, smell, and sound, as well as tension, pain, or pleasure are constantly sending signals to your consciousness. Sensations are a whole-body experience. They keep you in touch with your body—if you pay attention to them.

Senses bring valuable information from the outside to the inside. It's how your inner world knows what's out there—you see it, hear it, smell, touch, or feel it. Even though the world we see and touch is "out there," we actually experience it "in here," in our own place, through the nerve endings in our body and the brain waves of consciousness.

Because the direction of charging moves from outside to in (where discharging moves from the inside out), the senses play a big role in charging us up. We get excited (positively or negatively) from sights and sounds, smells and tastes, and someone's touch—all because it brings in energy from outside and stimulates the nervous system.

But *processing* this energy is another story. Nerve endings that receive sensation are literally all over the body—*100 million of them!* Yet there are *10 trillion synapses* in the nervous system itself, making the mind *100,000 times more sensitive to its internal world than to its external environment.* So we have a lot more infrastructure dedicated to *assimilating* sensation than to *receiving* it. Processing sensation must be pretty important!

In terms of evolutionary survival, the brain's ability to turn sensations into action is how animals avoided danger, whether through the sound of footsteps, the smell of an enemy, or cold air compelling a squirrel to store nuts for the winter. In mammals that have no cerebral cortex to figure things out, actions had to be based on how things *feel*. When something feels wrong, we pay attention and take action.

Yet, like survival instincts, most of our sensations happen below the radar of awareness. After a while, we no longer notice the tight belt, the noise in the background, or the ugly picture hanging on the office wall. We get so used to the heavy chest that accompanies sadness, or the chronic constriction that results from fear, that it becomes normal. But when we consciously direct our attention toward those sensations, they take us deeper into our feelings and emotions, needs and desires.

As sensations come into consciousness, they clump together to form *feelings* and *emotions*. You might say that sensations are the words, feelings are the sentences, while emotions tell the story—at least the story we tell ourselves. If my skin is crawling (a sensation), then I *feel* uncomfortable or wary. The *story* I might tell myself is that someone is out to get me, and the *emotion* might be fear or anger. So there's a whole continuum between the senses, feelings, and emotions.

Sensations, then, are the first key to unblocking emotional charge. They are also the key to grounding it, as they bring us into our physical tissue. If we were exposed to a lot of unpleasant sensations in the past, we shut down this channel of awareness. We numb out and bind our charge with habits that keep our awareness occupied elsewhere, like watching TV, eating, drinking, smoking, or keeping constantly busy. When we're numbed out, we become senseless and need "sensationalism" as a stimulus. Advertisers and news media use this regularly to entice the public, many of whom live with repressed emotions and blocked sexual charge. We buy products that promise to make us feel alive or sexy.

With our senses open, we can behave "sensibly" rather than being "senseless" or "insensitive."

Feelings and Emotions

As sensations come into the body and start to bring up charge, they gather into rivers of feeling. An underlying mood would be considered a feeling. You might feel optimistic, irritated, uneasy, or despondent. Each one has a characteristic sensation in the body. Irritation feels very different from apprehension or depression, which are all very different from optimism.

Emotions, however, are more focused and more highly charged. You are angry about this, sad about that. Ideally, emotions come and go, flowing like their watery element. We don't want to drown in our emotions, nor do we want to block them. We can feel our emotions deeply and express them authentically, without repressing or exaggerating our emotional charge. That's the healthy state, but for most people, it doesn't happen that way.

Too much charge makes it difficult to handle our emotions. We get swept up in the river of feeling, carried by its intensity. Too little emotional charge and we go through life mechanically, numb to our experience. Emotions also connect people. Too much can feel overwhelming and invasive to another, while too little can make someone feel flat, dull, and distant.

But what are emotions really made of? Sensations alone do not produce emotion. I can feel the warmth of a sweater or the coolness of air-conditioning, but it doesn't make me emotional. There are stories and beliefs associated with emotions, but the thoughts do not determine the emotions; they merely provide the context for them.

As feelings meet increasing charge of the body, they become emotions. Whenever charge goes through the body, it tends to heighten whatever emotion is there. All emotions carry charge, and charge usually (but not always) has an emotional component. In fact, the stronger the charge, the stronger the emotion. Fear and anger, for example, are known for having intense charge. Increasing our charge in those situations will make us feel more afraid or more angry. Joy and excitement are also states of high charge, states that we experience as pleasurable. Without freeing up our charge, we can't have the full pleasure of these states, nor can we maintain them. But our ability to manage our emotions depends on our ability to handle their charge.

Emotion, then, is an experience of charge moving through the body. The word *emotion* comes from the Latin prefix *e-*, meaning *out*, and *movere, to move.* While sensations move inward, emotions tend to move charge up and out of the body, from inside to outside. And once again, *feeling* an emotion brings up charge, while *expressing* an emotion is a discharge. If I feel sad, I can feel the charge of heaviness in my chest. If I have a good cry, I discharge the sadness and my chest becomes lighter.

The positive emotions are the "yes" factor—you like what is happening and want to make it continue, like being excited or happy about something. The negative emotions, such as fear, anger, or sadness, are a "no" response. They want something to stop or change. The body responds to this duality with movement— we draw toward what we like and push away from something we don't like. When emotions are blocked, so is the body's fluidity of movement. Likewise, when we restrict our movement, we restrict the flow of emotion.

Emotional charge originates in the gut, moves up the core through the third and fourth chakras, and then out through the mouth, hands, and eyes. When we start to feel an emotion, we often say, "Something is coming *up* for me." That's a natural path of discharge, and if you are helping someone release emotion, you want to open that pathway. This movement from below the belt upward to higher awareness is a movement from the unconscious to the conscious that makes us realize what we're feeling. When we repress an emotion, the charge has to become stronger in order to rise up into consciousness.

In addition to being felt, emotions generally want to be expressed or discharged. For infants and toddlers, who are too young to speak or take command of their environment, raw emotion is the best expression they have. When they feel something, they express it immediately and fully. They can cry like it's the end of the world when a toy is taken away and then be happily engaged in something else five minutes later, because they don't inhibit the discharge.

But we've all had to learn to inhibit our emotions to some degree. When emotional discharge is unavailable, unsafe, unwanted, or inappropriate, then the charge can get stuck in the second chakra or at any of the exit ramps, like the arms, legs, or throat. Since the element water implies movement and flow, blocking emotion results in *blocking the flow of charge in general,* resulting in a kind of rigidity, not only in the body but also in one's thinking or behavior. Then, when the charge does come up, instead of being felt as emotion, it goes into reinforcing the rigid defense. We will talk about that more when we discuss the Rigid character structure in Chapter 23. For now, just think of "keeping a stiff upper lip" as representing the stiffening that we have to do to repress emotion.

Present and Past

Past experiences create a groove for the river of emotional charge. They pave the way for emotional habits and the stories and beliefs we create to support them. If you experienced fear from a raging parent, you will be more afraid than your co-worker when your boss gets angry or critical. If you have a history of feeling rejected, you will have a stronger emotional reaction to getting dumped by your lover than someone who felt well loved as a child. Understanding the past can help you embrace your emotions from a place of compassion. But the charge that arises is here in the present. That's where healing takes place.

Unfortunately, most people ignore their charge and focus instead on their story. They go over and over the disappointing details or incessantly worry about what might go wrong. Instead, if you move the story into the background and focus on the sensations in your body, you move from "out there" to "in here." You come back to "your own place" in the present moment and begin the healing process.

When a client tells me they are feeling an emotion, I always try to track the sensation of that emotion, such as a clenching in the gut, rapid heartbeat, or tightness in the chest. Following the sensations is a way of tracking the charge and getting out of the story. I have them feel what the charge is doing, where it is trying to go, and where it might be blocked. By heightening and exaggerating the sensation at the edge of the comfort zone, as we learned in the Focus and Exaggerate exercise on page 51, we soften the blocks and the charge will start to flow again.

But what happens when you repeatedly experience a negative sensation, such as pain, tension, or unbearable heaviness? The emotional reaction—and its story—initially becomes more intense or insistent. "I hate this; I am scared to death; I am really angry." Or: "How could she do that? Why does this always happen to me?" The emotions naturally want to go to action. But if action is impossible, we use our energy instead to repress the emotion. Then we might find it harder to take action in general and wonder where all our forward movement went. Well, it got stuck in the blocked emotional charge!

When we can't take action to avoid an unpleasant experience, we have to numb ourselves to withstand it, and that means diminishing our sensation. Since charge heightens sensations in the body, we numb ourselves by stopping the flow of charge in general or by minimizing the amount of attention we give to our sensations. Then we become out of touch with our feelings and out of touch with ourselves and our own inner place. Without that barometer for sensing what's happening, we make bad decisions, override our emotions and live with the consequences, and then numb out even more to make do with the situation. Sound familiar?

Like the instincts, our emotional charge also arises beyond our conscious control; we don't "decide" to be afraid or angry—it just happens, often very quickly. What we *can* decide, however, is whether to contain the emotion or to express it—to hold it in or to let it out. That is, unless we lose the ability to maintain control, and then whatever gets stimulated is immediately expressed, much as it is with young children. But even as adults, I'm sure we all know some people who can't seem to contain their emotions at all, while others are so contained, they seem to show very little emotion.

Sometimes the action needed is simply for the emotion to be expressed and witnessed. Women know this well. Often they just want to shed their emotional charge and be heard. They want their emotions validated. And if they're not heard, they intensify the emotions, much to the chagrin of their male counterparts, who grew up repressing emotion. Somehow, when we get empathy, we feel less alone in our feelings, more able to cope. For many people, tears come on stronger when someone's listening than when they cry alone. The emotional charge has a way to connect with another being and can flow back and forth.

When it comes to positive emotions, we certainly don't want to repress those, but we do want to repeat them. If you have a wonderful time with a friend, you want to see your friend again. If you love the taste of chocolate, you're going to want to eat it often. These emotions move us forward; they "motivate" us—from the same route, *movere*, to move. But it's hard to be motivated if we don't let ourselves feel.

Limbic Resonance

Emotions are connected with the limbic system, an interior and lower part of the brain that is evolutionarily 100,000 times older than the cerebral cortex, our thinking layer. Sometimes called the *mammalian brain*, the limbic system governs our emotional well-being. It's highly connected to a part of the brain called the *nucleus accumbens*, which is the brain's *pleasure center*. This part of the brain plays a central role in sexual charge and the high that comes from recreational drugs.

When two people are emotionally in tune with each other, there is said to be a *limbic resonance*. That's a fancy term for what a child feels when they are held, nurtured, and protected by loving parents, just as it should be. When all is well, the limbic system hums along, creating a pleasant feeling. When disturbed, however, it dominates our attention until things get better and the disturbance is fixed.

Our sense of pleasure and well-being are heavily modulated by the limbic system's production of *dopamine*. Dopamine influences sexual arousal and gratification, and especially reward and reinforcement. (Pavlov's dog got a dopamine surge.) This means that when we get a reward, such as a pat on the back, a pay raise, a hug, or a cookie, the limbic system creates a surge of dopamine, and that reward can be addictive. It makes us want it again.

Dopamine plays an important role in motor control, hence motivation, which is why rewards work so well to motivate people. Dopamine makes us alert, while *serotonin*, another important brain chemical, helps us to relax and sleep. Both dopamine and serotonin pour into the *nucleus accumbens* pleasure center, one of the few places in the brain where both these chemicals meet.

When the limbic system is repeatedly disturbed, we may disconnect from our emotions partially or entirely. Disturbance is a rupture of limbic resonance that then triggers a variety of physiological responses in the body that all boil down to an arrested flow of charge. Charge that no longer moves, contrary to the fluid nature of the second chakra, becomes a blockage in the stream of consciousness. But it doesn't just block the negative experiences;

it minimizes our window to experience in general, blocking the pleasurable feelings as well. And it may bring our dopamine and serotonin levels out of balance, creating anxiety or depression.

When a child feels the charge of fear, for example, their limbic resonance is disturbed. Young children tend to go to a parent for comforting, and a responsive parent will hold them, bounce them on their knee, or stroke their back and speak to them soothingly. This restores limbic resonance and helps to regulate the nervous system's disturbance. When a child receives this regularly from his caretakers, the child learns to self-regulate his charge and maintains a healthy balance of charge and discharge.

Unfortunately, too many children fail to receive this regulation from their parents. Then the limbic system remains disturbed along with the sense of well-being. That feeling of disregulation may endure, even when there is nothing in present time to be upset about, because it's lodged in the body as an emotional habit. That means any time charge comes up, it can trigger reactivity or disregulation. And with that can come shame over one's feelings and more blockage of the emotional flow.

That doesn't mean the charge of the emotion isn't rolling around in the second chakra somewhere. It just means that your consciousness isn't very connected to it; the river is dammed up. When stimulated, however, by anything remotely resembling the original feeling, the emotion suddenly wakes up full of charge, rushing to be released. We've all experienced this when we get triggered by something our partner says and suddenly some emotion is up and running us, and we're helplessly carried along by it. The emotion is stronger than the situation warrants, because it touches into an old story and an old place of stored charge.

Emotional charge can also be stimulated by a sensation similar to the original experience, such as the smell of alcohol, a particular season, or the sight of an abuser's face. I remember once, long ago, a whole cascade of emotions arising because I heard a piece of music. It took me three days to figure out what it was connected to—a traumatic situation from my past—but my charge was through the roof until I made the connection. I knew of another person who was afraid of grass and flowers—an unlikely source of fear. In therapy, he recovered a memory of being a baby on a blanket in a field with flowers. Suddenly a cow stood next to him and licked him! That's traumatic to an infant, as the cow is so large and scary to someone that small without the motor capacity to run away. But the smell of grass and the flowers was enough to trigger the disregulation of his charge.

When emotions are triggered, they contain the charge of all the experiences that created a similar feeling. When someone dies, for example, it can open up the grief from all the losses in your life, from your childhood cat to the teenage boyfriend who dumped you to your lost opportunities. When anger is triggered, it can carry the charge of every time your brother teased you or all the anger you could never express toward your father. That can be a lot of emotional charge trying to get out the door. And because it's too much, we try to slam the door shut. Not that we shouldn't learn to contain ourselves, but there is a cost involved. The pressure builds up and either becomes pain in the body, numbness in life, or heightened emotion when the charge next arises.

Sexual Charge

While we get our emotional programming from our childhood, as adults this all plays out in the realm of sexuality, the crux of the second chakra. Here we find the lure of positive sensations, the need for emotional connection, the desire for limbic resonance, and the innate drive toward pleasure all rolled up together. In reflection of the duality of the second chakra, we also face the binary risk of acceptance or rejection at this most intimate level. Sexuality also involves movement—not just outer movement of the body but the inner movement of erotic charge, the desire to be met and satisfied.

Ideally this charge moves beyond just the genitals. Someone who is sexually open and reasonably turned on can feel this erotic charge move through their whole body. It's intoxicatingly pleasurable, and when we find it we want more of it. This is a charge that typically likes to build to a peak and then be released as orgasm, a pleasurable release of that charge.

Sexuality generally goes through a natural process of the charge–discharge cycle, discussed in Chapter 4. This keeps the second chakra fluid and balanced, releasing the old and letting in the new. The flow of erotic energy through the body not only puts us in touch with our body, it also nourishes the cells and the nervous system with new energy. Its release through orgasm brings relaxation and kindles intimate connection.

The healthy balance of sexual charge gives us an erotic connection to life in general. The sharing of touch literally puts us "in touch." When culture began to repress sexuality, an important connection to our bodies and to one another was lost, along with our sense of pleasure and well-being and a vital mechanism of balancing our charge. Our culture became out of touch and, as a result, I would argue, more violent.

Sigmund Freud called this erotic charge *libido,* though it meant far more than just sexual charge. Libido is really the flow of the life force in general, a basic biological drive. Without it, we don't have as much desire to do anything. But when sexual charge is blocked, it can also lock up our libido in general, and we have little energy or motivation to do anything. If we're not experiencing pleasure, then why would we want to?

When the body is bound up with blocked emotional charge, the erotic charge becomes blocked as well. Both take place in the realm of feeling and sensation, both relate to chemicals in the brain's pleasure center, both involve movement and release in the body, and both involve connection with another human being and all that person's charge as well!

Orgasm

The complete flowing back of the excitation toward the whole body is what constitutes gratification.

WILHELM REICH

So let's bring this all to a peak and talk about orgasm. Orgasm, as most anyone would agree, is a strong and pleasurable discharge. The stronger it is, the deeper the pleasure. If we review the chart on page 36 of the bell curve of charging and discharging, we see that a full discharge results from allowing the erotic charge to build to fullness and release, after which the ideal is to slide down into relaxation, with some intimate snuggling and then to fall sleep.

Premature orgasm is the inability to let erotic charge build to its fullness, while inability to achieve orgasm can be either failure to increase enough charge or a fear of releasing into the egoless state of discharge. Sexual addiction can be a way of binding the charge that doesn't release fully. If the release is only genitally focused rather than a whole-body experience, such as being on a porn site versus being with a real person, it can be addictive. Not only does it prevent a full-body charge through sensuous touch from another, it gives the sense of a reward that triggers an addictive dopamine response. But emotionally, it's safe, as it's not a real person.

When I lecture on these topics, people always ask me about masturbation. Is it binding the charge or releasing it? Is it healthy? My answer is that it depends on the attitude of the person masturbating: Is it a sensual whole-body experience or just a discharge of tension? Is it self-loving and erotic or self-loathing and cloaked in guilt? Often masturbation can allow one to connect deeply with their own place without the distraction of another. And when one is not in a relationship and has no lover, masturbation is a way to remain connected and open to one's sexuality and the pleasurable flow of charge and discharge.

So orgasm plays a huge role in the regulation of charge, through allowing discharge of energy, not only from sexual arousal but from the tensions of everyday life and emotions in general. Blessings on whatever creator gave us this function, for without it, other forms of discharge take over.

Researcher James Prescott has shown that cultures that repress sexuality tend to be more violent, while cultures that are more sexually permissive have less violence. He states: "As a developmental neuropsychologist, I have devoted a great deal of study to the peculiar relationship between violence and pleasure. I am now convinced the deprivation of physical sensory pleasure is the principal root cause of violence."[1]

We need only look at our world, and its rampant repression of healthy sexuality, coupled with systematized violence, through wars, movies, and media, to see how this plays out. The old adage of "make love not war" was actually grounded in fact.

Excess and Deficiency

When the second chakra is excessive, the emotions carry too much charge. People with this pattern tend to have a round, protruding belly, as if it has expanded to hold all that watery charge in there. The watery essence of the second chakra tends to spill over, leak out, or otherwise muddy things up. One may feel their feelings so intensely they have to express them immediately and strongly. The pressure of the excessive charge within wants to get out to become balanced.

However, if the pathways are continually used, as in someone who chronically rages or cries, those pathways will get reinforced whenever charge comes up and can become habitual, even addictive. It is important, when releasing emotions, to allow them to bring conscious information so that we can make appropriate changes in our lives and not have to relive the same thing over and over again.

When the second chakra is deficient, there is too little charge. Emotions are flat, the body is rigid, behavior is either self-controlled or controlling others, and sensation may be muted or numb. When the second chakra shuts down, so does one's sex drive, and we can lose our important orientation to pleasure. Deficiency can make for rigidity in the hips, stiffness in the joints, a flat belly, and rigidity in one's attitudes.

Excess and deficiency in the second chakra can sometimes be seen in the angle of the pelvis, deficient when the hips and pubic bone are pulled back, excessive when pressed forward. When someone is chronically swaybacked, it is likely they are not releasing their charge in this chakra. If their hips are chronically pushed forward, they might be unable to hold a charge or they might release charge prematurely.

Balance

Ultimately, balancing the energies of the second chakra bring ease and pleasure, grace and fluidity, a sense of being grounded in one's own experience, in touch with their emotions, yet not ruled by them. The second chakra receives charge, moves it through the body, and then releases it, keeping the body in balance. Then the charge can move on to the higher chakras, which we will visit in the ensuing chapters.

Pelvic Wave Exercise

Begin with the standing grounding exercise, summarized here, which is designed to get energy moving up from the earth into your legs and torso. (A more thorough description of the grounding exercise can be found under Opening the Leg Channels in the previous chapter.)

With feet shoulder width apart, pressing down and out, like trying to push the floorboards apart, inhale and bend your knees slightly. Exhale and straighten to about 90 percent of a straight leg, being careful not to straighten your leg all the way or lock your knees.

Once you begin to feel the tremble in your thighs, it's time to bring the charge into your second chakra.

As you inhale and bend your knees, press your tailbone toward the back, increasing the curve of your sacrum. As you exhale, push down and out through your legs while bringing the pubic bone forward.

Repeat both movements slowly, coordinating with the breath—pelvis moving back on the in-breath, forward on the out-breath.

While this exercise is more subtle than the grounding exercise, you will start to feel a bit of charge come into your pelvis. To help it move through the body, on the next exhale, as your pelvis thrusts forward, let your whole torso make a wavelike motion, starting at the hips and moving upward. Repeat many times and follow any natural or involuntary movements that arise.

Butterfly Exercise

Lie on your back with the soles of your feet together and your knees out to each side. (If this is uncomfortable for your inner thighs, you can support the outside of your knees with pillows, yoga blocks, or rolled-up blankets.)

Tune into your breath and find the natural movement of the breath through the spine. Notice the spine's natural arch on the in-breath and the natural pushing downward on the out-breath. Take several deep breaths here to feel this subtle movement.

Now we add the movement of the knees. As you exhale, slowly bring your knees together, pressing the back of the sacrum into the ground. As you inhale, slowly bring your knees out to each side, arching the small of your back. Allow your breaths to be long and full, and allow your movements to match the breath—one full opening of the knees with each inhale, one full closing with each exhale.

You can, however, experiment with speeding up both the breath and the movement and find the speed that most brings charge into your pelvis.

Stop when you can feel the charge in your pelvis, and just tune in to your own place. Follow whatever movements your body wants to do.

If by some chance you feel overcharged with this exercise, or it brings up uncomfortable feelings, I suggest you do some big movements with your whole body to discharge. Go for a run, dance, or jump up and down and shake it out.

chapter 13

CHAKRA
Three

|||||||||||||||||||||||||||||||||||||

Moving Anxiety and
Depression into Action

Sexuality and anxiety present two opposite
directions of vegetative excitation.

WILHELM REICH

In the third chakra, charge arises for the purpose of *action*. Whether it's action in service of survival, as it is in the first chakra; action in response to emotion or desire, as it is in the second chakra; or simply wanting to accomplish a task, the third chakra is oriented to *doing* something. This requires energy, which in the third chakra is correlated with the element fire. Generating that energy and directing it effectively is the task of this chakra.

Combining chakras one and two, you can see how energy is generated by the combination of matter and movement. You move a part of your body, such as opening and closing the palms rapidly as we did in the hand chakra exercise on page 7, and this generates energy in your hands. You go for a run, and you energize your legs. Yoga classes start with a warm-up movement to get your muscles energized.

Generating energy is the first step toward power. What we do with that energy is directed by *intention*. Intention originates in the upper chakras from consciousness. It begins in the mind and moves from the top down. You *think* that you want to practice yoga every day, or you *intend* to get that report finished by Friday so you can take the weekend off. We all know how many intentions we have in our minds. Without fulfilling them, they are just a thought. We might not have the time or energy that day, or we might be unclear on the intention itself, but too often they don't get fulfilled.

When intention coming down from consciousness meets the energy rising up from the lower chakras, they combine at the third chakra and move outward into action.

Mastery

When you successfully accomplish what you intend to do, you get a sense of satisfaction. Think of the way you feel when you cross something off your "to-do" list and turn it into a "ta-da!" It's a great feeling, like getting a check in the mail. Success builds the confidence that you can do it again, which in turn creates self-esteem and personal power, all of which are important aspects of the third chakra.

People who fulfill their intentions get results, and this creates a sense of personal power. If someone intends to work out four days a week and actually does so, he gets not only the satisfaction of following through but the results of a fit body. Results are a positive feedback system that builds power. Everything we create on purpose requires the ability to direct energy into our intention. The larger the intention, the more energy we need to fulfill it.

Ultimately, the goal here is mastery of your energy. A master makes what is difficult seem effortless. A master painter, for example, captures a likeness with a few brushstrokes. A master pianist lets the music flow through her fingers effortlessly. A master skater slides across the ice with twirls and jumps that look much easier than they actually are.

The ability to direct your charge into purposeful, skilled action is a mark of that mastery. To get there, it takes repeated effort and practice and usually lots of patience. But eventually, through all your hard work, the effort becomes effortless. That is mastery.

Mastery of the energy body means that you can allow your charge to build and still be able to manage it appropriately. You can increase or decrease your energy through physical exercises, which we will explore in this chapter. By working through your blocks, you can expand and embrace your charge. And through being clear and directed with your intentions you can accomplish what you set out to do.

When we don't *know* what to do, or when the desired action can't take place, the charge can get stuck in the third chakra area of the solar plexus. You may be unsure of yourself and therefore hold back, afraid of making a mistake, even sabotaging your success out of fear. Or your mind may give your will conflicting intentions: "I want to be recognized, but I'm scared to be seen." "I want to work more, but I want more time with my family." "I want to lose weight, but I want to eat what I want."

Any of these conditions can result in an imbalance of the third chakra's charge. We might feel a complete absence of charge, or we may feel the charge is simply blocked. In either case, it becomes difficult to do what we intend, and this diminishes our sense of power and self-esteem.

Anxiety and Depression

Anxiety and depression are hidden epidemics in western society. In the U.S. alone, *40 million* adults over 18 years of age suffer from anxiety disorders, or about 18 percent of the population. Yet this only reflects reported cases. Estimates of unreported cases brings it up to about one-third of American adults, with the numbers higher for women than for men.[1]

Worldwide, the average is much lower, 7.3 percent of the global population, though the World Health Organization (WHO) still considers anxiety one of the major health problems of the Western world.

Depression, at the other end of the spectrum, affects nearly 15 million American adults. It's the cause of two-thirds of all suicides, which incidentally outnumber homicides three to two (even though homicides receive a lot more coverage in the news). Women's rates of depression are twice that of men.[2] Globally, 350 million people of all ages suffer from depression.[3] These are alarming statistics.

At its simplest level, the excessive and deficient diagnostics of the third chakra are based on whether someone has *too much* energy or *too little*. Anxiety can be viewed as too much charge, while too little can feel like depression. Any treatment of these disorders needs to include mobilizing this blocked charge into action, guided by the intentions of higher consciousness.

While it's certainly important to ask, "What are we doing wrong in this society that's causing all this suffering?" such an answer would require a book of its own, if not several. But we tend to ignore the cause in favor of antidepressants and addictive substances. However, there are other ways to deal with anxiety and depression: *We can learn to mobilize our charge.* And when we do, we become more effective change agents for the world around us.

Anxiety

The root of the word *anxiety* is *angere*, which means to choke or squeeze. Anxiety is having too much energy moving through a constricted or choked-off space. When we create blocks, tense our muscles, or bind the charge, energy builds up. Just as a river going through a narrow channel turns into white water, energy flow becomes more intense when it's constricted.

High charge plus constriction equals anxiety.

Anxiety has certain sensations: we feel butterflies in our belly, our heart beats too fast, our mind races, or we can't sit still. We get many fits and starts toward action, but the action is blocked in confusion and self-doubt. Unable to spend the charge through action, it instead builds up in the body as tension.

Afraid of letting out this intense energy, we create even more muscular tension, which perpetuates the anxiety. This constriction keeps the charge from moving into action and actually intensifies it. The concentrated high charge paradoxically strengthens the constriction in a vicious cycle that one feels powerless to break.

Exercise (including yoga) is a treatment of choice for both anxiety and depression. Exercise increases endorphins (the chemicals that give you a high after a good run), as well as naturally producing GABA (gamma-Aminobutyric acid), which is a neurotransmitter that reduces excitability in the nervous system. People with anxiety are often low in GABA. In other words, they can't calm their nervous system.

The key here is to befriend the charge and allow it to move through your body, into a *discharge*. If you jump up and down, shake your arms wildly, and make loud sounds, you are helping your body release charge. Better yet, go for a run, put on lively music and dance and yell, or clean your house. *Simply doing something—almost anything—will help.* Getting rid of some of the excess charge will bring the level down to a more manageable size. Then the body can relax its constriction, and the result is feeling calmer.

If I'm working with a client who is constricted with high charge, I often have him push into my hands while I put up resistance, giving him something to push into. I encourage the client to make sounds as he pushes. I let him do a small amount of discharge, then pause and wait to see what the body does. Invariably, something settles in the person. He calms down, breathes deeper, and feels more relaxed and present. I may need to do this several times to bring the client back into his comfort zone, but each time moves him toward a feeling of relaxation and spaciousness.

If you're alone, however, you need to find something to push into. I suggest the following exercises.

Doorway Push

Stand in a doorway, with your feet over the threshold. Bring your arms to the side and press your palms into the doorjamb on both your right and left at midtorso level. Push down into your feet and simultaneously outward into your hands. Take a few breaths as you push, lengthening the exhalation of each breath, even with a sound. Then slowly release your hands and bring them over your solar plexus. Notice your breathing. It is probably slower and calmer, while your hands may feel warm and energized.

Stand Up and Shake

The simplest technique to discharge is just to shake yourself out. Stand upright on both feet and begin to bend and straighten your knees, such that you bounce up and down a bit, without your feet leaving the ground. Once you start the movement, get your arms and hands involved. Add your voice, making abstract sounds, or even words if saying something arises naturally. Let it get to the point where the movement is happening by itself. Shake until you feel your charge level come down.

Woodchopper

This exercise begins in a wide stance—with your feet planted about three feet apart. Grounding firmly into your legs and feet, clasp your hands together and raise them up over your head. Imagine you are holding an axe between your palms. Allow your back and belly to arch just slightly. Take a few breaths and let your energy build, like a cat getting ready to pounce.

When you feel somewhat charged, take a breath in, then on the exhale, make a loud "Ha" sound as you swing your arms forward and down, as if you were hitting a chopping block with your imaginary axe. Then rise up again and repeat several times, allowing the whole body to move in one smooth release, and making sure your "Ha" sound is loud and forceful. Practice with different sounds, especially with the word *no* or even the word *yes*. When tired, return to standing and pause, noticing what your charge feels like.

Depression

Like the freeze-or-fold phenomenon of the first chakra, the third chakra can also collapse or implode, meaning the energy moves inward against the self, instead of outward into action. Without energy and power to meet the challenges of life, everything feels overwhelming. This seeming lack of energy undermines the will and weakens motivation, focus, and follow-through. Without these essential third chakra skills, the repressed charge fuses together disappointment with failure, victimization, and self-blame into a complex that spirals down into depression. Once this complex takes hold, it becomes self-perpetuating, which is what can make depression feel so hopeless to those who suffer from it. When depression is severe, even basic actions, like getting out of bed, taking a shower, or going to work become difficult.

The word depression derives from the prefix *de-*, meaning *from*, and the word *press*, which reflects the way consciousness from above *presses down* against the energy that is naturally rising up the chakras. Afraid to take a wrong action, we don't even allow the energy to arise. Compare this to the previous discussion of intention and energy working together as will, and you see that in depression the energy is held back by a downward current that is stronger than the upward current. It's not that we don't have intentions. It's that the energy rising up from below is not strong enough to overcome the resistance, inertia, and negative thoughts that arise in consciousness.

Of course, depression can originate from very painful circumstances, especially those that seem to have no solution. Exploring childhood issues and the lessons of the past can help to understand the depression, which certainly helps with the self-judgment, but it usually doesn't fix it. While I don't wish to minimize the suffering people have gone through, the point of mobilizing our charge is to get those things behind us instead of in front of us, blocking our way.

Sometimes in depression the will becomes so disabled, it's no longer connected to the self at all, meaning we respond more to the wishes of others than to our own desires. While that may make us into a doormat for others—at least on the surface—unconsciously, the will goes into a kind of rebellion—what I call *outer compliance and inner defiance*. Outwardly, we are going through the motions, but inwardly we are resisting, which is like driving with the brakes on. This takes more energy than necessary and wears us out over time, only adding to the lethargy and depression. We'll learn more about this pattern when we study the Endurer character structure in Chapter 21.

Anger is a fiery, powerful charge. It wants to take direct and immediate action. Alexander Lowen, founder of Bioenergetics, said that anger was a charge that went straight up the back, holding the body upright. Without that charge, we don't have enough "backbone" and the body slouches or collapses. Not that it's healthy to be angry all the time, but when anger is habitually blocked, it hits a wall in the front edge of the third chakra and turns back against the self, often as a vicious inner critic.

Earlier, we saw how matter and movement produce energy. Alexander Lowen has noted, in reviewing videos of working with depressed patients, that they only make about half the spontaneous movements of nondepressed people, and in some cases, hardly move at all.[4] Without generating energy through movement, the body doesn't have enough charge to throw off the internal suppression, and the result is defeat and despair.

When the backbone is activated, it holds the torso upright, allows the lungs to expand, and gives room for the digestive organs, all of which contribute to a healthy, inner fire. I have often seen digestive issues, weight problems, and depression clear up when someone accesses and releases their anger in a safe way. By *safe*, I mean expressed in a way that does not cause harm to oneself or another. Pounding a pillow, saying (or yelling) what needs to be expressed, or writing a letter that is never sent can all be ways of releasing anger safely. Some people are afraid that if they do that, it will turn them into an angrier person, but in most cases I find the opposite to be true. Once the anger is released, they actually become softer and less likely to get triggered.

Exhaustion, from putting out so much energy over a long period of time, can also lead to depletion and depression. When exhausted, we need to extend our comfort range be able to tolerate being at a low charge level long enough to deeply relax and rest. Deep rest allows the charge to build again. People who are busy all the time, constantly doing things, tend to be afraid of those deeply relaxed states. Then, when the exhaustion hits, they reach for more stimulants to keep going, rather than allowing themselves to rest. This depletes the adrenal glands and leads eventually to a deficient third chakra.

If depletion is a result of exhaustion from too much discharge, or simply from too much work or stress, we need to rest. Using exercises to regain our charge when the body needs rest is like drinking coffee to stay up all night. While it may work in the short run, it robs the body of what's really needed. But if depression is a chronic state, even after rest, then we can do some practices to generate energy.

As with anxiety, if you're depressed, you need to get out and do something. Easier said than done, because when one is depressed, getting motivated to do something is the hardest thing in the world. Then you need some simple techniques to bring your charge up. Once you have some energy to work with, things are not as difficult.

Generating Energy

Depressed or not, we all like the feeling of having enough energy to get things done. The ubiquity of coffee shops shows just how many people want to feel more energized. Why, I just had a cup myself prior to sitting down to write! And while there's nothing wrong with that, we can also generate energy by pushing charge through the body, including the limbs, as well as by tapping on certain points and getting the body moving.

When I teach about the third chakra in my workshops, it often comes at that point in the afternoon when everyone's energy is low. After I talk about the third chakra and tell people we're going to get up and do some vigorous exercises, I look around the room, and people look back at me like I'm crazy—like it's the last thing they want to do. I promise them that after we're done they will feel much more energized, and I'm always proven right. So if you feel depleted and these exercises seem daunting, have faith: you will feel better later.

Three Thumps Exercise

Donna Eden, author of *Energy Medicine: Balancing Your Body's Energies for Optimal Health, Joy, and Vitality,* suggests a simple practice called the Three Thumps[5] to wake up the body. This practice takes only a few moments and can be very effective.

1. Press your thumb and first two fingers together, making a kind of pointed beak.

2. Then gently thump or tap on the points shown in the diagram on page 153 10–20 times each, starting with the points under the clavicles (K27) and ending with the spleen points.

She generally recommends following this with the Cross Crawl exercise, to get the right and left sides of the body working together optimally, as a way to balance one's energy. This exercise begins in a standing position.

1. Place your weight onto your left leg and lift your right knee and left arm simultaneously upward.

2. As you bring them down, alternate by lifting your left knee and right arm.

3. Continue back and forth several times.

4. I like to tap my hand to the opposite knee before lowering my leg each time. This is also a good alternative if you are unable to stand for any reason.

DONNA EDEN'S 3 THUMPS

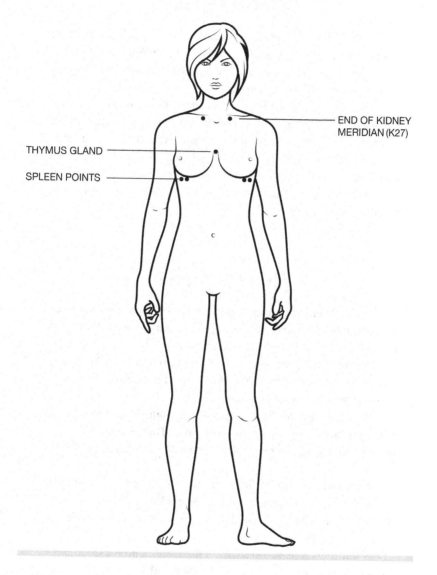

END OF KIDNEY
MERIDIAN (K27)

THYMUS GLAND

SPLEEN POINTS

Figure 9 Three Thumps:
Tap on these points to generate a more energetic state.

Punch Out

Begin with the Stand Up and Shake exercise on page 148. Even though this is listed for anxiety, it works for depression too, as it begins to shake off the imaginary straitjacket that's holding you down and gets the energy circulating.

Next, imagine you are punching into the air in front of you. Make a fist in each hand, and alternate between your right and left hands punching forward on the out-breath. I used to stand a futon on its end for my clients to give them something to punch into, so if you have something soft to punch into, great, but otherwise the air will do. Using sound will increase your breath, which in turn builds up your charge.

Breath of Fire

This is an energizing and purifying breath from the yoga tradition. It can be done anytime and anywhere you feel you want to perk up your energy and strengthen your core.

Sit comfortably with your spine erect, your crown chakra placed directly above your base chakra. Place a hand over your solar plexus, between the navel and the breastbone.

With your mouth closed, rapidly snap your diaphragm inward, forcing a quick burst of air out your nose. Then simply relax your diaphragm and notice how the air comes back in by itself. That is one round.

This exercise repeatedly snaps the diaphragm in again and again, forcing the exhalation while allowing for a passive inhalation. Start slowly and build up speed as you gain skill at this exercise and develop your belly muscles.

A few rounds of 40–50 snaps of the diaphragm is a good place to start. Stop if you feel dizzy and simply breathe naturally.

Act from Choice

When desire and will are aligned, energy moves more freely. We have more charge when we *want to* do something than when we *have to*. We have more energy to get up early to go on vacation than we do when going to work, for example. If we are inwardly telling ourselves, "I have to do this, I have to do that," we will undermine the body's natural enthusiasm, and our charge becomes dull and plodding. Too many "have-tos" are depressing.

Changing your inner dialogue from *have-tos* into *choose-tos* enlivens your will. If you can't find any reason to choose something, then see if you can find a way *not* to do it and choose that. We could say we pay our bills because we have to, but we can also reframe our inner monologue to say we are choosing to pay our bills because we want to keep our credit in good standing or to keep the lights on. We do the dishes because we are choosing a clean kitchen.

Reflection Exercise

Make a list of the things that you don't want to do, yet tell yourself you have to do them.

List the reasons why you are choosing to do those things. Answers might include pleasing someone else, wanting to look good, or needing a certain result.

If the reasons are important to you, then make it a conscious choice to do those things. If not, consciously choose to say no.

Exercise Your Brain

Establishing new brain circuits, especially when they involve physical as well as intellectual learning, can be very helpful in alleviating depression. Tackle something new, like playing an instrument, learning a new language, studying dance or yoga, or engaging in a new sport. Even a change in scenery can help, or having a stimulating conversation that opens new ideas.

Practice Gratitude

It's easy for a depressive person to look at the negative side of things. Studies show that keeping a gratitude journal and writing down things you are grateful for each day stimulates the anterior cingulate cortex in the brain (the place that connects the old, primitive brain and the newer prefrontal cortex) and helps regulate serotonin and dopamine imbalances, as well as reducing insomnia.[6] Rick Hanson, in *Hardwiring Happiness,* suggests that it is natural for the mind to focus on the negative. We counteract that with a conscious practice of really savoring the positive experiences we do have, which rewires the neural circuitry of the brain to experience more happiness.

Examine Your Beliefs

If depression comes from consciousness pressing downward against the vital energy, then one usually has a number of negative beliefs operating. Often depression is accompanied by a belief that something is hopeless and will never change, limiting beliefs about oneself, or negative beliefs about the world. It's easy to find evidence to support these beliefs—that is child's play, as these beliefs began with our experiences as a child. What's more productive is to create beliefs that are uplifting. If you find your negativity is too strong to actually believe something positive, try pretending. See what it would feel like to *imagine* a belief in a positive outcome. Run that fantasy through your body and begin training your body to carry the energy signature of a positive belief.[7]

Work with the Cause of Depression

Generally speaking, we learned to depress our energies long ago, during childhood. While it's beyond the scope of this book to analyze all the many messages and traumas given to children as they develop their energies, it's worthwhile to examine the milieu in which power and energy were held in your family of origin. What were the teachings you received about your energy and actions? How were you treated as you were developing your will? Were there consequences to taking action that made you afraid to do so? Was there more expected of you than was appropriate for your age at the time? Were you seen and valued for who you are?

The power dynamics in your family can have a positive or negative effect on your third chakra. Uncovering these unconscious programs and making them conscious is the beginning to changing them.[8]

Excess and Deficiency

Excessive third chakras have too much energy and gravitate toward power and control, which, when blocked, turns into anxiety. In extreme, such a person can use their will to dominate or bully others. More commonly, it is simply the need for control. But another form of third chakra excess can be constant doing and the inability to retreat and be quiet and still. In this way one is dominating their natural need for rest and relaxation, with the power of the third chakra excessively running their lives (and often the lives of others).

Deficient third chakra people are afraid to take their power. They have trouble setting boundaries, being assertive, initiating, or following through with their will. They may be tired and lethargic, unable to find their vitality, and find themselves falling into depression.

Balancing the Third Chakra

If you don't have enough energy, you need ways to generate it. We generate charge in the body through good diet, breath, movement, and rest when necessary. Getting the body moving in general, whether through yoga, walking, or something more vigorous like dancing or aerobics, will mobilize trapped charge, stimulate the metabolism, and, over time, create a more fit body that runs charge more effectively. Ultimately, it requires doing practices with regularity to make a permanent change. Once you spend more time in a better state, it becomes easier to maintain that state. Doing these exercises for both charging and discharging will free up channels for charge to move. Notice how you feel as you do these practices. More important than some kind of formula, find what works best for you to feel balanced.

chapter 14

CHAKRA
Four

||||||||||||||||||||||||||||||||

Opening to Love and Intimacy

At the touch of love, everyone becomes a poet.

PLATO

There's nothing like that feeling of falling in love. The flow of charge is exciting and uplifting. Everything glows with light and significance. Food and sleep seem unnecessary. We even say we're walking on air—an apt metaphor, since air is the element of the heart chakra. Air is expansive and soft, without boundaries. Air describes the lightness of the heart when it's full with the charge of love. We crave that feeling, just like we crave breath.

The charge of love is basic to our well-being. To a child it's essential, perhaps the most powerful form of charge that we receive. The love from caring parents gives the child comfort when she is scared or hurt, which teaches her to regulate her own charge. Whenever someone gives us their loving attention, we receive a gift of charge and fill our vessel with the inner glow of love.

But when love is taken away—either through rejection, loss, betrayal, or the death of a loved one—there is a tremendous crash, as the charge level drops dramatically. The energy implodes around the heart chakra, sinking the chest. We lose not only the person, but a major source of charge that has come through their love. Such is the feeling of grief—what I call the "demon" of the heart chakra—a feeling that is antithetical to a light and happy heart.

Grief sits on the heart chakra like a stone. It brings heaviness and constriction, where the element air is light, expansive, and free. When grief strikes the heart, ancient hurts and betrayals, past rejections and losses—everything that hasn't been properly grieved—comes up again, along with all its unexpressed charge. The ancient rejection from your first boyfriend or girlfriend, the loss of your dog 10 years ago, and the end of your marriage all mix together in the painful tenderness of the current loss.

The good news is that releasing that grief cleanses the heart chakra and lets it shine forth once again with new light, much as the sun looks brighter after a good rain. Not that it's an easy process—facing the reality of pain and loss is always difficult. But if the charge behind the grief can be released in its full, chest-heaving sobs, the grief passes more quickly.

The Balance Point

Love is simultaneous mutual regulation,
wherein each person meets the needs of the other,
because neither can provide for his own.

FROM *A GENERAL THEORY OF LOVE*

The heart chakra is literally the "heart" of the whole chakra system—the midpoint—with three chakras above and three below. Its symbol is a 12-petaled lotus with two intersecting triangles— matter coming into spirit, and spirit coming into matter, perfectly balanced. Therefore an essential attribute to the heart is *balance*: balance between upper and lower chakras, between mind and body, inside and outside, giving and receiving, will and surrender.

Imbalance creates pressure. If there is more charge on the inside than the outside, the excess energy wants to get out and be freed. We feel a pressure to express, to do, to discharge. If we can't do that, we might feel anxious.

But if we're depleted on the inside and the charge is higher on the outside, we feel the pressure pushing in on us. The result is overwhelm and collapse, what the previous chapter described as depression.

When charge is truly balanced, we don't need to defend against what's outside, nor do we need to inhibit our expression. We can relax. Balance brings peace, equilibrium, and ease. We are centered in our core, open to the exchange of energies between our inner and outer worlds.

Relationships are a prime place where we try to balance our charge, from the first exciting thrills of flirtation, to eventual love-making, to the deepening of affection or the activation of arguments. Like everything in life, the flow of charge between two people fluctuates, never remaining static. If the overall balance of charge within a relationship can be maintained, the relationship tends to last. If it's unequal, it cries to be addressed—usually by the one who feels shortchanged. If the imbalances cannot be addressed, the relationship erodes and becomes dysfunctional, or comes to an end.

While it's a bit oversimplified, I could say that most of the issues that couples have brought to me over the years can be boiled down to an energetic inequality. "I initiate sex more than she does." "I'm the one who's always trying to communicate." "I'm the one who is more responsible." "She's too emotional." "I do the lion's share of taking care of the kids and the housework." "I'm the one providing more of the finances." It usually boils down to one person feeling like they are either giving too much or not getting enough in return.

We have talked about how living organisms function best when there is a balance between charge and discharge. When the body is open, meaning unarmored, then the charge is free to enter and leave the body organically, without having to think about it, just like the breath balances itself between inhalation and exhalation. When the heart is open, we neither cling nor push away because we have access to our own source of charge. But when we have to defend against unwanted energies coming in from outside, or by contrast, protect the vital energy in the core from coming out, we lose that balance. Then we armor the heart.

Armor, by definition, is hard. If a soldier goes into battle, he needs his armor to be hard and impenetrable. For just about everyone, at some time or another, life has been hard. To survive, we had to harden our hearts, and often our bodies as well, a habit that became part of our permanent structure. When we armor the heart, or any other part of the body for that matter, our defended state becomes normal. We can't take the armor off, even when we want to, and often we don't even know it's there. Usually, it falls to an intimate partner, who bumps into that armor, to point it out. And when they do, they trigger all the stored charge buried behind it, often with a barrage of defensiveness.

The key to opening the heart, dissolving the armor, and coming into balance is *softening*. As we age, we harden, become stiff and rigid, and lose our equilibrium. Think of a baby, who is naturally soft, and a child, who is still softer than an adult. If our boundaries are soft and permeable, energy can more easily pass in and out. We experience this naturally when we sleep, which is perhaps one reason why we wake up refreshed, yet tender and vulnerable.

Exercise:

Softening Meditation

Close your eyes and bring your attention to your inner world. Find your alignment by pressing your roots downward, into the earth, and lifting your crown upward, toward the heavens. Feel the central column of energy, your core, running vertically between crown and base.

Once your vertical alignment is established, bring your attention to your breath. Allow your breath to slowly deepen, taking in more air on the in-breath and letting out more air on the out-breath. Notice that the breath is soft; it doesn't have any edges or boundaries.

Allow yourself to wait after each exhalation until the urge to inhale comes naturally, to wait at the end of each inhalation until the urge to exhale comes naturally.

Imagine that someone is gently putting a hand on the back of your heart chakra, giving you support, while gently pressing your heart slightly forward and upward.

Imagine now that the air around you is a field of universal love and that every breath you take fills you with that love and every breath you let go of contributes to that field of love.

As you breathe, soften your chest, your shoulders, your lips. Soften your arms and hands. Soften your legs. Imagine that the boundary between inside and outside, the boundary of your skin, becomes very soft and permeable—that you can breathe in and out through the pores of your skin, love coming into every pore, love releasing through every pore.

Imagine softening your stance on an issue. Maybe you soften toward another person in your life, or maybe you soften how you regard yourself. Imagine that this softness allows you to return home to your innermost self, where the inner beloved resides. Imagine this inner beloved as a field of love, radiating and shining out into the field of love that surrounds you in a perpetual exchange of love, compassion, and forgiveness.

When you are ready to open your eyes, open them with a soft gaze that allows you to remain connected to yourself and connect to the outside world at the same time.

The Breath

Deeper breathing creates deeper feeling because it creates movement from within, and movement enables feeling.

JOHN STIRK

In relation to its element air, the heart chakra can be accessed through the breath. An exuberant heart takes a full breath, and a closed heart inhibits the breath. Breath is energy, and the more air you take in, the more charge you will have, while shallow breathing results in less charge and lower energy.

Many people unconsciously inhibit their breath to avoid the feelings that increased charge might bring up. A child who experiences repeated negative feelings numbs herself by keeping her charge low and will subconsciously hold the breath in order to do so. Extreme fear also freezes the breath, probably a carryover from needing to be quiet and remain hidden. Fear can also leave you in a chronic hyperarousal of fight or flight, which makes you breathe faster and may result in overcharge or anxiety.

The breath is inhibited by rigidifying or hardening the muscles around the chest. This may begin as an act of self-protection, but over time it becomes unconscious armoring and a closed heart. When armoring is dissolved—and I know this from countless sessions, both receiving and administering therapy—one of the first things that happens is that a person takes a deeper breath. This is an organic process that happens by itself when healing takes place. A deeper breath allows expansion, which gives you more room to have your charge.

While opening the heart invites us to naturally take a deep breath, we can work that principle in reverse: we can unlock the heart through practicing deeper breathing. In deepening the breath, however, the charge of past emotions may rise up to consciousness again, to be reexperienced and released. Holotropic Breathwork, which is intense, rapid breathing for an hour or more, brings up these intense emotions that have been buried. Ideally, the emotions that arise can then be released.

Most emotional discharge, such as yelling or crying, happens on the out-breath. When emotional feelings are present, but their expression, or discharge, is not permitted, then one has to inhibit the exhalation. I have always believed that a primary cause of asthma comes from not being allowed to cry. Asthma, in turn, may be activated by deep crying, intense exercise (which requires deeper breathing), or the presence of noxious substances in the air (such as cigarette smoke).

Without the ability to discharge, we cannot let go, return to a lower-charge, relaxed level, and make room for something new. In the heart chakra, that means we have less room for love.

Breathing Exercises

The Winged Breath

The Sufi tradition often depicts a heart with wings, indicating the expansive nature of the heart. You can think of your arms as the wings of the heart: they reach out, they expand and contract, and they are connected to the muscles around the ribs and chest.

In this simple breath, you inhale and expand your chest, opening your arms wide, spreading them like wings. As you exhale, round your chest and bring your hands inward, giving yourself a hug. Feel yourself cradling your own heart.

As you inhale again, allow your chest to lift upward and expand forward, once again opening the arms out wide.

Repeat several times, allowing your body to follow with any other movements or sounds that spontaneously arise.

Then stop and notice if your charge has shifted in some way.

Twisting Breath

This is an energizing breath that will bring charge into the heart chakra area. The breath comes in through the nose and out through the mouth.

Sit in a comfortable upright position where you have a bit of space around you to move freely. Place your hands on your shoulders and hold your elbows out to the sides at shoulder height. Breathe in through the nose and twist your upper body to the right, allowing your head to follow the movement, looking over your right shoulder. Then quickly twist to the opposite side as you exhale through the mouth, again allowing your head to follow the movement, looking over your left shoulder.

Repeat 12 times, breathing in to the right, breathing out to the left.

Then center yourself and switch to breathing in on the left and out on the right, as you repeat 12 times again.

When you stop, take a moment to be still and feel the charge that the breath brings into your upper body. Make note of any feelings that arise.

Alternate Nostril Breathing

This exercise is a basic yoga breathing practice (*pranayama* to balance the breath, calm the mind, and soothe the nervous system). It is excellent for balancing the left and right hemispheres of your brain and for creating peace and equilibrium.

Sit comfortably cross-legged or in a chair, with your spine comfortably erect. If you are in a chair, make sure your legs are uncrossed so that your hips are level and that your feet are on the floor.

With your right hand, fold the second and third fingers into your palm, extending your thumb and ring fingers. Take a deep breath. With your right thumb, close off the right nostril and exhale fully through the left nostril. When the breath is empty, breathe in once again through the left nostril.

When the breath is full, use your ring finger to close off the left nostril, and exhale through the right. Inhale again through the right, and when the breath is full, use your thumb to close the right nostril again, breathing out and then in through the left.

Always switch nostrils at the top of the breath, meaning when the breath is full. Breathe out and then in again through the same nostril. Breathe slowly and deeply. Practice 10–20 rounds of this breathing, and then sit quietly in meditation for a few moments or longer.

Vulnerability and Intimacy

While most people crave intimacy, they often fear vulnerability. Unfortunately, we can't get one without the other. What is it that makes us feel vulnerable? And what is it about vulnerability that makes it so difficult?

Vulnerability usually comes about when we are expressing something intimate about ourselves, something that has a fair amount of charge. If it didn't have any charge, it wouldn't feel vulnerable! But when we truly bring the inside out, especially regarding matters of the heart, the blocked charge tumbles out along with it. We may cry or shake, or the voice may tremble when we're sharing something important. It's that release of charge, I believe, that feels so vulnerable. We don't know if the other person will receive it openly or react by closing down against us, criticizing, or otherwise withdrawing in our moment of need.

Of course, if you were not allowed to release emotional charge growing up, this is going to feel even more vulnerable. Men, who are trained by the culture to not be emotional, often have a harder time being vulnerable, but this is certainly not limited to men, nor does it apply to all men. We all have a hard time with this.

When the deep charge inside does come out, it wants to be met, witnessed, and accepted. It wants to be loved. When what is inside us meets another's insides, that is intimacy. An open heart can meet another in their vulnerability and isn't afraid to be vulnerable in turn. An open heart creates and sustains intimacy.

Electromagnetic Charge in the Heart

So far, we have been talking about charge as something that we feel in our bodies, as an arousal of excitement, intensity, or sensation. But there are subtler kinds of charge as well. As we climb up the chakra column, we move into subtler levels of energy, so the heart is an important place to move from the big actions of chakra three to the subtler currents in chakra four.

There are direct neural pathways from the heart to the brain, specifically to the part of the brain called the *amygdala,* which is part of the limbic system. The amygdala serves a central role in our emotional reactions, as well as processing emotional memory and making decisions. It's interesting to note that the left and right amygdalae perform slightly different functions: the right processes positive emotions such as joy and happiness, while stimulation of the left amygdala produces the more negative feelings of fear and sadness.[1] In addition, the left amygdala is more active in social anxiety, PTSD (post-traumatic stress disorder), obsessive-compulsive disorders, and borderline personalities.[2]

There is even a term coined by Daniel Goleman, author of *Emotional Intelligence: Why It Can Matter More Than IQ,* called the "amygdala hijack." This is a fancy term for when emotional triggers "hijack" our thinking part of the brain and produce a reaction out of proportion to the actual situation. When this happens, the high charge is running without the modulation of the brain's reason, and we can say or do things we might later regret.[3]

While this may seem more connected to the emotional level of the second chakra, the reason I bring it up here is that the cells at the core of the amygdala *synchronize with the heartbeat.*[4] It seems that the heart's rhythms inform the amygdala and influence our emotional state. Incoherent rhythms can be interpreted by the amygdala as cause for anger or stress, while coherent rhythms indicate that things are copacetic.

The HeartMath Institute has done some fascinating research into the functioning of the heart, not just as an organ but as a coherent field of radiant, electromagnetic energy, a field 5,000 times stronger than that of the brain. A central aspect of their research focuses on the phenomenon of heart resonance or coherence. They suggest that states of inner harmony, peace, and well-being correlate to coherent patterns in the rhythms of the heartbeat. They state:

"In essence, because the heart is the most powerful biological oscillator in the body, when its rhythms are 'in tune' with the natural resonant frequency of the heart–brain communication system (i.e., in a state of coherence), the amplitude or amount of heart rate variability becomes greater. When this happens, the heart rhythm can pull and shift other oscillatory systems into entrainment and synchronization with it."[5] This results in an overall state of well-being, harmony, lowered blood pressure, and relaxation.

HeartMath's Freeze-Frame Process

This simple exercise can be done very quickly to combat stress, sadness, depression, or anxiety by developing great heart coherence. When you notice you are feeling stressed or anxious, begin by taking some time out (even a few minutes will do) to disengage from the thoughts that are causing you stress by doing the following:

Focus on the physical area of your heart chakra (heart, lungs, chest, and upper back areas).

Imagine that you can breathe in and out through your heart chakra, taking several deep, slow breaths.

Think of a positive experience from the past—a time when you felt love for someone or loved by someone, a time when you were content, safe, cared for, etc. If you cannot remember a time, then make one up. Let that feeling radiate through your heart and the rest of your body. I tell my clients to imagine "soaking their cells" in the experience.

Spend a few breaths here, noticing any changes.

Excess and Deficiency

A highly charged heart chakra is so full of energy that it radiates outward toward others. That energy may be loving and supportive, uplifting those whom it touches, or it may become co-dependent and meddling, out of touch with its own center.

While it may be hard to imagine how we could have an "excess" of love, remember that an excessive chakra is the result of a *compensation strategy* rather than a full and happy chakra. One who did not get enough love growing up might compensate by needing to be the center of attention, by excessively focusing on their social life, or by having poor boundaries in regard to others.

A deficient heart chakra, by contrast, has shut itself down, isolating from others, becoming critical, cold, and judgmental of self or others. A deficient heart chakra is locked in self-protection, but it locks out the very love that it needs. Boundaries may be too solid, whereas an excessive heart chakra can exhibit very weak boundaries.

Ultimately, what we need is balance. As we soften our bodies and reduce the armor of the heart, that balance begins to occur naturally in the constant give-and-take that is the perpetual reciprocity of love.

chapter 15

CHAKRA
Five

|||||||||||||||||||||||||||

Speaking and Handling the Truth

Words are the language of the ego in the same way that movement is the language of the body.

ALEXANDER LOWEN

Nearly everyone has experienced what it's like to have charge caught in your throat chakra. That sudden cat-got-your-tongue feeling when you can't seem to speak, the way your voice gets small and tight, or a chronically tight jaw are all symptoms of trapped charge in the throat area.

This chakra correlates with the element of sound and represents your ability to receive, assimilate, store, and express communication. Here in the neck, at the meeting point between the head and the body, the charge is so palpable—you can see and feel it immediately when it's there. *That's because the throat chakra is one of the main places of discharge.*

I remember the clients who came to me for body-oriented therapy yet wanted to yak their way through the whole session, using a torrent of words to bypass their body or emotions. And I'm sure we all know someone who never seems to shut up, much to the annoyance of everyone around them. Still others are perpetually quiet, having trouble speaking up even when they want to. In my workshops, nearly everyone feels like they have some sort of block in the throat chakra.

In the second chakra, we looked at how the senses are gateways where the outside comes in. The fifth chakra, by contrast, is where the inside comes out. In other words, I don't truly know what's going on inside of you unless you tell me. Whenever you open your mouth to speak, you let the inside come out. That can be a very vulnerable thing to do.

Of course, we do have superficial conversations where we don't let out much of anything that's inside, such as giving instructions at work, lecturing on an academic topic, or making small talk. These kinds of conversations don't carry a lot of charge. In fact, many people stay entirely within this superficial level, simply because it's safe.

Speaking Your Truth

When you speak your truth and allow the inside out, it's often accompanied by a backlog of stored charge—as if all that charge has just been waiting to find an open door through which it can escape. If you've been holding something back for a long time—some truth you've wanted to say to your partner or a story from your past that you've never told anyone before—a tremendous amount of charge can arise when it finally does come out, even more charge than the situation warrants. This makes the essential purpose of communication—to share information about what's inside—obscured by the intensity of built-up anger, tears, criticism, or fear.

For this reason, such communication can become scary, unwieldy, or too hot to handle. If you're a person for whom communication wasn't safe growing up—and that includes most of us—or if you're at work, where it isn't appropriate to share your truth, then you have to keep the inside from coming out. But when the gate is open, all that charge wants to rush out the door, and we can totally overwhelm the other person. They look at us and say, "Wow, where is all that coming from?" Our charge is then running us instead of us being in charge.

The opposite can also happen. We can unconsciously constrict the throat chakra, making even simple things difficult or scary to communicate. I've seen it happen many times in therapy when a charged topic comes up; the voice suddenly becomes small and tight, almost like a child's voice. I can actually see the muscles around the throat and chest tightening and the breath constricting. It's in these moments that we need to stop the words and drop down into the body and really feel and listen to our internal charge.

Sometimes it can help to do a little discharge through the voice, hands, and feet, so that it's not all trying to get out the mouth at the same time. Push into something solid, like a desktop or doorway, and make abstract sounds, such as grunts and moans. This helps discharge the excess so you can get back to your truth without having to handle all the additional charge.

When we do express our truth—and it's heard fully and responded to with empathy—the charge seems to level out. There's an internal satisfaction that settles into the body. We go "Ah," and that torrent of energy that's trying to get out slows down. We've spoken what's important and heard an answer. We feel met. A communication cycle is completed. The charge is balanced and neutralized.

But too often, communication is less satisfying than that. We try to say things but can't find the words. We feel we're not listened to, or we feel misunderstood. We try again to get our point across, and the charge starts to escalate. As it escalates, it becomes even harder to communicate.

When someone is coming at you with a torrent of words accompanied by strong charge, they are unable to listen until they have discharged what they have to say. Unfortunately, most of us are busy trying to get a word in edgewise when we're in the face of intensely charged communication: "No, that isn't so. You don't understand. I need to say this. You're not listening!" It falls on deaf ears, because the capacity to receive is blocked by the outpouring of charge through the throat chakra. Once a person has discharged, he or she is more able to take in new communication.

Stephen Covey, in *The 7 Habits of Highly Effective People*, said, "If you wish to be understood, seek first to understand."[1] Once the other person feels understood and heard, they are more ready to hear and understand what you're trying to say. It's a difficult practice, but well worth the effort.

All communication has at least some charge. If you are trying to say something and it has no charge, it probably won't be heard. I know in my own life, my trouble saying *no* comes up in this regard. Sometimes something will happen, and I'll say to myself, "I know I said *no* to this." But I realize I didn't say it with the full charge of conviction, so it wasn't heard or taken seriously. I often work with clients to strengthen their *no* by pushing against me with their hands and saying *no* until I feel the word has its full charge and really lands on me.

So if all communication has charge, I would venture to say that when we are afraid to speak out or to hear a truth, it is because *we are afraid that we can't handle the charge of it.* We may be afraid of our own charge coming out, or we may be afraid of the other person's charge in reaction. But whatever is not expressed then becomes charge stored and locked up in the body. It's like it hangs out in the print buffer, and as soon as you charge up the system, like turning on your printer, it spits out that document you were going to print yesterday. We may find ourselves saying things we regret or wondering how *that* came out of our mouth—why, I sound just like my mother!

Vibration and Communication

Imagine that the central channel of your core, along which the chakras are located, is like a vertical string. When the energy of the core is extended downward, into the earth, and upward, toward the crown, the two ends of the central line are stretched out like a string on a guitar. When life plucks that string, as it surely will, it vibrates in response. That vibration lasts until the strength of the impact on the string is canceled out. On a guitar, if you hit the string hard, the sound is louder and lasts longer; if you pluck it gently, the sound is softer and shorter.

As I have shared in my Hay House book *Chakras: Seven Keys to Awakening and Healing the Energy Body,* anything that impacts us—whether it's as simple as someone bumping into us on the street, or a more impactful experience, like the loss of someone important—the impact vibrates this vertical cord of the soul. Small impacts, like the noise of trucks passing by and phones ringing, have an effect too, but they are largely ignored because they're so commonplace. Still, if we're exposed to them all day long, we will feel stressed at the end of the day. Just notice the relaxation and relief that you feel when some background noise, like a lawn mower or a fan, finally shuts off, and you realize we're more influenced by sounds than we think.

More powerful events, such as getting fired from your job or hearing about some terrible tragedy, make us want to talk about it—which is a way to *vibrate that impact back out until it is neutralized.* We come home from work and want to say to someone, "I gotta tell you what happened to me today!" We want to get that information off our chest. And we feel better when we do—if we are received and understood. Even a therapist whose only skill is to be a good listener can do at least some good by allowing her client to get things off his chest that have been held in for years or decades.

So when the impact upon our soul is vibrated back out, the charge settles back down to normal. We are then ready to be plucked again—meaning we have the ability to listen and respond to what's around us. I'm sure we've all been in a conversation with someone where we were so busy with the voice inside our own heads that we didn't really hear what the other person was saying. That's because this chakra was simply too full. Until we release some of what's in there, we don't have much capacity to listen.

What Blocks Communication?

If it's natural to express what impacts us, what happens when we can't do that? What happens to the child who can't tell anyone what happened at school or can't tell their teacher they are being abused at home? What happens when a child speaks and isn't heard, isn't believed, or is shut down and made to feel wrong in some way? What happens when a child has to lie to survive, or is told to believe lies that contradict their experience? What happens when there are secrets in the family?

Then we create the habit of holding back our voice and shutting down the throat chakra. This shuts down the ability to communicate in general, just as it shuts down creative expression, confidence, and connection with the world around us.

In a guitar, if you pluck a string but don't want it to sound, you hold your finger on the string to keep it from vibrating. Guitar players call that "deadening a string." When we can't let something out that impacted us, we basically *deaden ourselves* and deaden the vibratory capacity of our body as a human instrument. This shuts down not only our communication but also our listening and creativity.

Unblocking the Throat

The purpose of the fifth chakra is to find the harmony and resonance of fully living and speaking your truth. The closer you get to your truth, the closer you get to the core vibration of your soul. That brings harmony and alignment and ease, while not being in your truth brings lack of ease, or even dis-ease.

Often, we don't even know what our truth is. Or our truth might be mixed: "I want to be closer to you, and I want some space right now." "I want to be seen and I have a need to hide." "I love you and I can't stand you sometimes." I find it is essential to speak these mixed truths, to not expect it to land on one side or the other. By saying whatever we *do* know is true, we begin to peel back the layers of deeper truths. A good conversation is like that. It has a way of deepening into ever more real and vulnerable truths, and brings people closer.

Of course, that doesn't mean we blurt out our truth whenever it suits us, or that we speak it out hurtfully, without regard for some guidelines on healthy communication. Small things, such as speaking in an "I" voice rather than "you," promotes more compassion and empathy. Saying "I feel scared when your voice gets loud," rather than "You are so angry and abusive to me!" or "I get annoyed when appointments don't happen on time," rather than "You're so disrespectful the way you're late all the time." "You" statements tend to put someone on the defensive, whereas "I" statements invite empathy. "I" statements are the inside coming out.

Guidelines such as Marshall Rosenberg's *Nonviolent Communication* or the Harville Hendrix Imago Relationship Therapy model for compassionate listening are very helpful for learning to communicate with skill and compassion and to communicate in a way that gets you the results you want.

Withholds

What happens in a relationship when we don't speak our truth? There is a word for all that we hold back, and it's called, logically enough, *withholds*. Whenever you have withholds from someone, it creates distance between you and that person. If you have a friend, an intimate, or even a work relationship in which there is a pile of things that haven't been said, you will find yourself feeling more distant from that person and likely more judgmental.

Here's a process to remediate that, one that unloads the throat chakra, gets rid of the withholds and lightens up the space and frees up the charge. It has a very specific set of rules, and it's important to follow these rules closely, as they create safety.

Speaker: I have something I have withheld from you. Are you willing to hear it?

Listener: Says *yes* or *no.* If *no,* the speaker can ask if there is a better time or if that means never. *No* must be respected or renegotiated.

If *yes*, then proceed.
Speaker: Last night, when you were out late, I was worried that something happened to you.
Listener: Thank you.
Speaker: And when I heard you come in, I no longer felt worried, but then I felt angry that I hadn't heard from you.
Listener: Thank you.

Sometimes withholds can go back and forth between the two people, each sharing one at a time, or sometimes one person can share several and then give the other person an opportunity to share their withholds.

The important point is that the "thank you" is the *only* response that the listener gives. They don't defend, agree, disagree, explain, or respond. They simply say, "Thank you." They are basically saying, "Thank you for sharing this with me."

Many people wonder if this creates problems on down the line. Does someone wake up in the middle of the night, thinking about what their partner said to them earlier? Sometimes this can happen, and if so, that can be the subject of a further communication at a later time. More often, what happens after the negative communications are expressed is that more positive communications surface. The result is that the two people feel closer.

Balancing Charge in Your Throat Chakra

We balance charge in our throat chakra with a variety of techniques. When the throat is really locked up, it can be helpful to start with abstract sound. Simply moving the body and letting out sounds or even simple words can bring tremendous relief. It can also take what is held in "off the top of the pile" so that deeper truths can emerge.

The next step up from making abstract sound is writing in your journal. Here you can safely discharge what's inside, using any kind of language you want, without worrying about hurting anyone's feelings. It can work just like withholds and help you discharge negativity so that you can get to what's positive.

The next-biggest step would be to practice communicating with a third person. Women know that talking to a girlfriend is a great way to discharge and process what we are feeling. This is not to condone harmful gossiping, but there is benefit in just having an ear to listen to you.

The most difficult step (because it has the most charge) is to communicate your truth with the actual person. If he or she is not alive or is unwilling to listen, you can write a letter, and that can help discharge. If you have first discharged through any of the previous activities, then you have less charge when you talk to the person in question and are less likely to say things you regret.

What about when someone is undercharged in the throat chakra?

Then perhaps the person needs to hear something instead of speak something. Often with clients, there is a tremendous settling of charge when they hear someone say things like, "You're safe now." "You didn't do anything wrong." "You're okay just the way you are." Or especially, "I'm sorry." These statements have powerful charge that often land right where they need to and bring about greater resonance and harmony within the body, emotions, and subtle energy. In my workshops, we often form a circle where each person gets a few moments in the center while the whole group chants a phrase of the person's choosing, such as the statements just mentioned.

Fifth Chakra Exercises

Get off My Back

Here's a simple bioenergetic exercise to loosen the area around the neck and shoulders, especially in the back body.

Stand with your feet at least shoulder width apart. Bend your elbows, and make a fist with each hand.

Begin, one elbow at a time, alternating left to right, moving the elbows rapidly toward your back, saying aloud, "Get off my back!"

After alternating back and forth, finish with pressing both elbows back at once. If any other words besides "Get off my back," wants to be expressed, feel free to do so.

Then stand and notice if your shoulders feel lighter and you feel more grounded.

Pressing on the Jaw

When we restrict our self-expression, we often tighten our jaw. This can create tension in the whole body. This exercise can be done by yourself but is more effective when someone does it to you.

Stand up straight with a nice wide stance. With your mouth closed and your head level, place your hand (or a friend's hand) directly under your chin. Then try to open your jaw, pressing against the resistance of the hand. Make a sound as you do so.

If making sounds is frightening for you, at first practice just the movement. Then add a soft sound and gradually increase the volume as you become more comfortable.

Excess and Deficiency

In the throat chakra, excess and deficiency are pretty simple. We either have too much to say or too little. We may talk more than we listen or listen more than we talk. The balance of input and output is tilted in one direction.

The throat chakra is one of the main avenues—and the one most accepted—for charging and discharging. If we consider how the neck is the narrowest part of the body between the base chakra and the crown, then it's easy to see how charge might get stuck in this "bottleneck" of the chakra system. Balancing charge in this chakra can pay off in better communication, enhanced creative expression, and better learning and listening. It can also create more connection between the head and the body, between self and other, and more harmony in your life.

We balance this chakra by expressing the truths found at our deepest core. We may not always get the answer we want, but at least we have cleared the chakra by speaking and releasing what's in there. That leaves room for more freedom, better listening, and more expression.

The Sanskrit name of this chakra is *Vissudha,* which means purification. When we release all that is stored in our throat chakra and clearly communicate our truth, we are purifying the subtle vibrations of the throat chakra. As the energies of vibration become even more subtle within the realms of sound, we find the resonance of our truth at deeper and deeper levels. As we embrace these truths, we begin to "see" more deeply as well, and this brings us to the next chakra.

chapter 16

CHAKRA
Six

||||||||||||||||||||

Charging Your Imagination and Vision

Imagination will often carry us to worlds that never were.
But without it we go nowhere.

CARL SAGAN

Now that we are moving into the upper chakras, we enter the more ethereal realms of mind and spirit. Here, at chakra six, located in the center of the head at brow level, we open to intuition and imagination. We learn to focus our attention and truly see the patterns within. To keep our gaze steady, we develop the neutral witness, creating a still place in the mind. As these aspects come together in what is also known as the third-eye chakra, we ignite the imagination and use the power of visualization to direct our charge.

All of this relates to the element of light—a higher and faster vibration than sound. It is only through light that we see. Seeing the outer world allows us to understand what's out there and how to navigate through it. That's an important kind of seeing, but one that we take for granted. Our deeper focus here is to cultivate the more subtle inner light that allows us to see inside ourselves, leading to *insight,* or sight within, and eventually illumination!

The name of this chakra—*ajna*—means to perceive and to command, reflecting both its passive and active aspects. Most of our seeing is passive—we just open our eyes and receive images of what's in front of us. Intuition opens through a receptive process of emptying the mind and allowing images to form. But *what* we see is a result of where we direct our attention. If I look out the window, my attention goes to the landscape. If I look at these words on the page, my attention is directed toward their message. If I am asking a question internally, my intuition is directed toward its answer.

We may not have a choice about what our eyes meet around us, but we do have a choice about where we direct our attention. In today's world, everything competes for our attention—every billboard, commercial, e-mail, and text message. Without a potent ability to focus, this can be distracting and lead to a scattering of charge. When we can focus all our attention in a single direction, our sight becomes like a laser beam, able to cut through illusion. By training our attention and calming the mind, our perceptions deepen.

Imagination

Using this chakra for healing and awakening involves a more active process of commanding our reality through conscious imagination and creative visualization. We imagine the results we want and thereby focus consciousness in that direction. We can imagine white blood cells clustering around an infection, a wound closing, or a bone mending. And while imagination itself may not be enough to warrant complete healing, it begins the process of directing charge toward that end. Where the attention goes, the rest of the energy tends to follow.

Imagination is a powerful force. It can generate potent charge, both positive and negative, depending upon the content. If you imagine lying on a beach with your loved one, you get a pleasant, relaxed feeling. If you picture getting rejected on a job interview, you might feel discouraged. We can get excited or scared, sexually aroused or turned off, simply by the inner picture we paint with our thoughts and attention. Positive or negative, however, these pictures exist only in our imagination.

Too often, our imagination has a mind of its own. We may get so lost in fantasy, we fail to see the reality that's right in front of us. We chronically replay negative scenarios or stare out the window in daydreams, when we should be paying attention to the here and now. It behooves us to look at how imagination, memory, and fantasy *command* our charge, reflecting the active part of the *ajna* chakra, to command. Turn your imagination toward more positive outcomes, and you begin the process of creating them.

Memory and Charge

I once lived with a housemate who had a negative image of herself. When she did something positive, like tidy up the kitchen, I would compliment her. But when she forgot to close doors or gates, I would point it out. In discussions with her later, she only remembered the criticisms, not the compliments. Her negative image was a filter for her memory. That's pretty typical, actually, as the brain tends to focus more on what's wrong than what's right, as an old survival mechanism. But it has its cost, for it can direct the energy into a negative spiral.

The pictures you hold in your mind direct your consciousness. They are the filters through which you receive and interpret your experience. If you think men can't be trusted, you will be more likely to interpret a man's actions as untrustworthy. If you think women are unavailable, you will interpret their busyness as proof that they aren't interested.

Both positive and negative experiences from childhood are stored in memory, along with all their attendant charge. When a memory is recalled, all its original charge can resurface, often very quickly. I know from my decades of sitting with clients that a painful childhood memory from 40 years ago can bring up as much emotional charge as if it happened yesterday. So too can positive memories of the past bathe the nervous system in an experience of relaxation, peace, or contentment.

In fact, memory and imagination are very similar to the body, with the exception that memory is often more familiar, because it actually happened. It has a deeper groove. But even when we revisit a memory, it isn't really happening in the present moment. It's just a reconstructed fantasy of what happened. And we all know that some memories have more fabrication than others, which is why two people can remember different truths about the same event.

So why do we remain stuck in negative memories when a good fantasy might bring us more pleasure? *Because memories from the past contain charge that is still seeking resolution.*

When any elements of a complex are triggered, such as a memory or a feeling, all the rest of the elements surface as well. This is a great opportunity to work with and heal the movement of charge through your body.

It all begins with developing the inner witness.

The Inner Witness

Your goal is not to battle with the mind, but to witness the mind.

SWAMI MUKTANANDA

Looking out through your eyes, hearing sounds through your ears, and experiencing life through your body, there dwells a quiet, internal awareness. This awareness is not your mind, which may run endless chatter, commenting and analyzing everything around you. It is not your body, which experiences pleasure and pain. It is not the rise and fall of your emotions, nor is it the images or sounds you see and hear. It's the part of consciousness that can perceive all of this. It's the part of you that observes.

Even while you react emotionally and your charge runs through your system, the inner witness is always there, whether or not you're aware of it. This witness is essentially neutral. It exists beyond all your value judgments of likes and dislikes, good and bad, right and wrong. Like a camera or a voice recorder, it simply sees and hears what's there. Our mind then interprets, judges, values, and analyzes what we experience.

Brain science teaches us that "neurons that fire together wire together." That means that the more you follow a certain thought process or habitual behavior, the more your brain molds itself around these patterns. When it comes to riding a bicycle or driving, that's a good thing. Once we learn, it's always there. But this principle also works in reverse, with negative thought loops, involuntary fantasies of doom and gloom, and bad habits. The more charge we run through these thought patterns, the more they run our lives.

The witness is something that exists behind all that. It is the part that can notice the thoughts you're having as if you were watching a documentary television show. *The witness has no charge on any of it.* It simply observes the nervousness, sadness, irritability, dread, or whatever else is going on inside you—*without judgment.* That is a key piece, because judgment tends to bring up charge. We get excited about what we like, sad or angry about what we don't like. And, of course, nowhere is this more evident than in judging ourselves.

As my students and clients continue to work with this material, I notice their increased capacity to witness their charge. They tell me, "I'm now noticing that when I confront someone, my charge comes up in my belly," or, "When I feel misunderstood, my charge races to my neck and jaw." The witness is simply reporting. "I'm noticing my charge is high and getting more intense in my chest." "I'm noticing my charge is fleeting, sometimes here and sometimes gone." We want to develop more of that capacity—*without having to do anything about it.* This means we can observe our charge without having to block it or discharge it.

Let's say somebody is rude to you and you feel the charge of anger. If you get triggered, the witness takes a back seat and a younger part takes over the driver's seat, and says, "She's so mean! I can't do anything right. She doesn't appreciate me!" Some other part of us—usually a younger part—is driving the situation, and we don't really know why. *The witness has been hijacked.* But the witness, with less charge and more neutrality, would say, "Oh, this person just raised her voice at me, and I notice a charge in my belly and throat."

Without this awareness, charge grabs our attention away from the witness. And then the mind makes up stories and interpretations about what happened. "You never listen to me. You don't respect me. You're so controlling. You don't care about my feelings." I'm sure we're all familiar with those little things we think. But are we able to *notice* we're thinking them, without getting caught up in their meaning?

If possible, let your witness observe the inner conversation. "Oh, this is what I'm telling myself." Notice your charge: "Wow, I have a lot of charge around this, and here it is in my chest. Here it is in my belly. Here it is up in my head, and I can't think straight. Here it is in my throat, and I want to babble, or I want to scream, or I can't talk because I have a block in my throat." The witness is noticing and saying, "That's interesting. I wonder what else I can learn about that."

So the witness is the part that can see clearly but detach from the charge. We're acknowledging it, but we're not in the middle of it. It is neither repressed, nor do we get caught up in it. And we might even be able to see multiple perspectives. "Oh, maybe this person isn't mad at me, but they just had a terrible day, or maybe they're letting off some steam from something in their past."

Develop the Witness Exercise

Sit comfortably in a position of meditation. Close your eyes, deepen your breath, and soften your body.

Imagine you can project your consciousness to a vantage point up on the ceiling, or even outside, where you can look down at yourself. You might be watching through a telescope or the lens of a camera.

Engage your witness, through your imagination, to observe yourself going through a typical day. See yourself waking up, and notice how you wake up—what are your first thoughts in the morning?

See yourself getting out of bed, taking a shower, getting dressed, eating breakfast, interacting with others.

See yourself going to work, doing what you do all day. Notice your conversations, your body positions, your thoughts and feelings as you watch yourself go through your day.

See yourself coming home at night, interacting with family or pets, or being by yourself, eating, relaxing, going to bed.

Notice especially anything about this person that she might not be seeing as she goes through her day. Notice what she is *not* noticing. Simply observe without judgment.

When you are ready to end the meditation, write down a few things that you observed that you might like to tell that person. Maybe you notice that they think they are more alone than they really are. Or that they could be nicer to people, or that they are not remembering that spirit is behind them.

What would it be like to go through your day with that awareness?

The Importance of Stillness

When charge is running us, it is difficult to be still. As we do our work of charging and discharging in the lower chakras, we begin to find equanimity, tranquility, and stillness. Just as a glass of muddy water that sits still for a while becomes clear, clarity results from being able to cultivate stillness in mind, body, and energy. This is best achieved through meditation, especially those practices that give the mind a single-pointed focus, such as a mantra, an image, or concentrating on your breath.

It is said that the sixth chakra is the place where dualities collapse into what we call non-dual consciousness. Dual consciousness is where one part of ourselves is experiencing life and the other is running an inner commentary about our experience. "What a nice day . . . Oh, but we need rain . . . Gee, she looks friendly. I wonder if it's okay to talk to her . . . Gosh, how much longer 'til lunchtime?" "I wonder if he's going to call me."

Non-dual consciousness simply experiences, without commentary. This is very difficult to do when the charge hijacks our attention and begins running our interpretations and stories. But if we have done our work rising up the chakras, refining our charge as we go, the whole system becomes quieter, yet remains alert and attentive.

Working with Charged Memory

When you feel charged by something, first look inside to see what got you triggered. I got triggered last night, for example, as I was getting ready to go to bed and my partner was texting on his cell phone and not connecting with me. It took me a full 10 minutes to even notice I had a charge around that, but as I climbed into bed, I was aware of being irritable and distant, even a bit snarky. So I tuned in to my witness and asked, "When did I start to feel this way? Oh yeah, just about ten minutes ago, when he was texting." Then I can say to myself: "Okay, this is here just to stimulate my charge so I can find out more about where I block it and how to let it free." And that is a different perspective than getting caught up in the stories or feelings. I can then notice where the charge goes in my body and where I block it, and use tools to harvest it, rather than make up stories that increase my charge. If I need to speak about the issue, I can do so with less charge.

As you feel your charge, step back for a moment to see what images come up in your mind. Allow yourself to free-associate with those images. *Just notice.* Let your witness report from a neutral place: "Oh, I see. That reminds me of when my mother didn't listen to me and she was so busy with all the children." "It reminds me of a past relationship when I found out he was having an affair." Or "It reminds me of how I often feel unimportant." Just notice the images that come up and look at them with a detached curiosity, as if you were watching a movie.

One trick that I find very helpful for remaining detached is to develop the capacity for *amusement*. When charge has a hold on you, either your own or somebody else's charge, being in an inner state of amusement seems to break the trance. If you find that you are constantly running the monologue of an inner critic, be amused when you catch yourself doing it. "Oh, there I go again, making myself wrong or bad. Wow, I sure do that a lot. Same old thoughts, over and over. Can't I even be original? How amusing!" Or, if you're on the phone with your mother and she begins to run her usual guilt trip about how you never do this or always do that, simply switch into private amusement within your own mind and allow the witness to observe: "Oh, there she goes again; now she's going to say that I don't call enough. Yep, that's exactly what she did. And now she'll tell me how much she sacrificed for me, and how my brother calls her more often. Oh, this is amusing." Amusement can break the hold a situation may have on you and give you the detachment you need.

Amusement is one aspect of this process. Another technique is to imagine a different interpretation that is more positive and then to imagine a different outcome. When your mother does her guilt trip about how you don't call often enough, you can make the interpretation that she loves and misses you, and this is her way of showing it. When harvesting the charge into your vision of a more positive outcome, it is important to bring that charge into the whole body. When my clients are visualizing something positive, I say, "Soak your cells in this." Notice how it feels to harvest the charge into your tissues, and savor that feeling, even as you visualize the outcome you want. This begins to build up a more positive base in the unconsciousness from which to operate.

Steps to Detach from Charge

1. When you feel charged, look to see what got you triggered. Be responsible for your own charge. Own it, and don't put it on the other person.

2. As you feel your charge, look inside to see what images come up. Look at them as dispassionately as possible. What are you telling yourself about them? What is your interpretation?

3. Find a way to self-soothe or harvest your charge.

4. Imagine a corrective experience.

5. Soak your cells in it.

Seeing Your Way Through

Seeing is an act of creation. If the root of imagination is "image," then we can further break down the word image to become "I" and "mage." Therefore, when the self creates an internal image, it is an act of magic.

Every time we go to manifest something, we utilize our imagination to direct our attention. If I'm looking for a parking place or a jar of spaghetti sauce in a grocery store, I imagine what I'm looking for until I see something that matches. I know what an empty parking place looks like, and I know what the aisle of jars looks like where I'd find spaghetti. The act of imagination directs my attention. When intention and image line up, we know we are on the right track. There is a kind of satisfaction that happens. "Oh, there it is." The charge settles.

Sometimes it's difficult to see our way through. Sometimes we are looking for something we've never seen before. Sometimes we find just the right thing, but it doesn't always look the way we thought it would. But always, what we see and imagine directs our attention, and where attention goes, the energy flows.

Develop the habit of imagining your day ahead of time. What kind of day do you want? How do you want to show up? How do you want to treat others? What do you want to accomplish? See your intention as if it were already so, and the command center will begin to create it.

As you develop the witness, you hone the powers of observation. The next step is to consciously create what you would like to see—creating a larger vision to guide you in your life. As your charge becomes more available to you—more under your *command*—it becomes possible to direct your charge into a vision of your choosing.

Simply imagine where you want to be next month, in a year, or in ten years. Imagine this every day, until it is manifested. Imagine little things, like the outcome of a conversation, and big things, like what you want your life to stand for. Make this a habit, and you will begin to take command, not only of your charge but of the course of your life.

chapter 17

CHAKRA
Seven

||||||||||||||||||||||||||||||||||||||||||||

Divine Consciousness
and the Charge of Beliefs

The most comprehensive work with the soul concerns its embrace of what we think of as the unknowable.

JOHN PIERRAKOS

Just as your laptop can connect with the Internet, where there's a vast storehouse of information far greater than your computer can hold, we, as energetic beings, can tap into an infinite field of energy far greater than our amazing little bodies can hold.

Such is the nature of the Divine: expansive, intelligent, and infinite. We can call it God, Goddess, Source, or whatever word we like, but it's not a theoretical concept; it's not a thought or an idea; it is a living, dynamic force of energy that exists within everything, enlivens everything, and from which everything is made. Take this energy away, and things would cease to exist.

The reason why we want to clear all the blocks in our chakras is to make more room to embrace this divine energy, for when it barrels through the body in full force, it can be almost too much to bear, wonderful as it is. Even so, we can never embrace all of it, but that's the nature of the mystery that lures us to seek the Divine.

When we begin to see everything as energy, as an emanation of divine force permeating the present moment, the whole world looks completely different. It's no longer an assemblage of things. It's not cogs in a wheel. It's not an array of cells, bones, and organs. It's not even people and animals, or nations, even though all these things do exist. It's the constant creative emanation of energetic patterns, rising and falling, interacting and dancing, that is the essence of divine reality.

Sometimes I think of it as clouds. If you lie back and look at the clouds on a breezy day, you'll see a little puff come out of this cloud and join another cloud. It's constantly shifting and exchanging. And in the same way, the whole universe is an exchange of energy. Some parts are giving energy, some parts are receiving, some are transforming, absorbing, or releasing energy. Some parts, like stars, are concentrations of energy. Like our sun, they beam light and energy into matter, bringing it alive. But it's all an intricate dance of energy.

And really, the closer you look, the more you see there are no objects. As we get down to the subatomic levels, there is no substance. It's mostly empty space conducting an exchange of energy. But it's not just energy *per se*. Wires conduct energy; batteries deliver energy. An explosion is a whole lot of energy. But are any of these things God? Do we experience the Divine when we turn on a flashlight or plug in a lamp? Typically, no.

In the seventh chakra, we learn to cultivate a deeper awareness of charge as the movement of the Divine in your soul. The story or situation that brings up your charge is simply the vehicle through which your life force is ignited within you. Ultimately, that charge wants to be freed from its limitations to return to its source in the infinite, back to the Divine once again. You might say the Divine is *wanting* to be freed inside you from all the places where you lock down against it. The Divine wants to awaken you, to take you back to your holiness, to your full flow of the same energy from which the universe is made.

So if your charge is an emanation of the Divine, would you want to get rid of it? Again, the emotions, the story, and the situation are just divine intelligence devising a strategy to bring it all up for you. So don't squander that gift by holding it in your gut or by blowing it all out in a burst of anger or emotion. Treat it like gold. Treat it as if the gods themselves have come to visit. Harvest the charge into your tissues, and allow your awareness to fully embrace the charge that you are.

This is the ultimate point of it all. To fully embody the Divine isn't to pray about it, talk about it, or read it in scripture. It's to allow this potent force to run through you, to fully live into it, to surrender to its power. But that surrender isn't a meek bow of obeisance, completely letting go of individual will. It is a living covenant between the finite self and the infinite Divine, between mortal and immortal. It is here that the Divine creates and manifests—through our very selves.

Stepping-stones to Deity

Let's take a quick review of how charge flows through the chakras to see how it plays out in the upward journey of the liberating current, traveling from the base chakra to the crown.

At the first chakra, we have the earth plane as solid matter. Every tiny atom that we can't even see contains enough energy to form a nuclear bomb. That's a lot of energy. But that's how great the potential is in matter. So the Divine is densely *stored* in matter, like energy in a battery. It's stored, but it's not free.

Energy is stored in matter for our use. We can burn wood, eat food, and build power plants out of wires and coils. Matter, you could say, is energy's intelligence, a manifestation of consciousness in form. When we push into matter, it's like plugging a socket into the wall. That begins the process of drawing energy out of matter—paradoxically by pushing into it. As we learned in chakra one, we do this by pushing our legs into the floor or earth, bending and straightening our knees slowly (see page 124). Whenever we engage with something solid, we create an exchange of energy, and that starts the ball rolling.

In chakra two, we begin to *move* the energy. From the base, it moves upward toward the opposite end of the spectrum, seeking freedom from its containment in matter. Once we plug in and we get energy moving through our hips and sacrum, we let ourselves *feel* the charge. In fact, we feel it *because* it is moving. Just like the second chakra's element, water, charge wants to flow. It wants to *go* somewhere. When we allow the charge to have a current or flow, solid matter melts into rivers of movement, distributing that charge through the whole body in subtle channels the yogis call *nadis.* The central channel, the *sushumna,* flows right up the core, from the base to the crown.

In chakra three, the power chakra, we begin to cook that charge, relating to its element, fire. Heating brings transformation, just as eggs, flour, and milk become a cake through the process of cooking. And here, we concentrate the flow into the *center of our charge,* the vertical column of energy that energizes the chakras. That turns the free-flowing rivers of charge into power, just as concentrating electricity through wires turns random electrons into power.

After focusing our charge into power, we can then allow it to *expand* in the heart. We allow this expansion by softening. We can't get to the Divine by contracting, even though that is a necessary stage to make the charge potent enough to rise up the spine. Eventually, we must move toward expansion to reach the infinite.

As the charge expands, we constantly refine it. We listen, attune, and purify our energies accordingly, alternately holding back and letting go. Now the charge becomes a subtle vibration, a deep, resonant hum of the soul's unique expression. The charge becomes the music the Divine is playing through the instrument of our lives. Going through the "bottleneck" of the throat area, that charge wants to again expand from expression to vision, from sound to light.

In the sixth chakra, we "see" the charge as a luminous light within and around everything. Patterns and images dance from the unconscious mind as hunches, intuition, inner visions. Through insight, or seeing within, we know how to navigate. We *see* the way.

But *who* is aware of all of this? With what are you aware? The journey to the seventh chakra is the awakening of the Divine within, as intelligent awareness. In that state, we realize that it's not only our own self that is aware, *but everything around us is also aware*—the trees, the mountains, and certainly the people, plants, and animals. They are all intelligence and energy enfolded into form, then unfolding according to an even higher intelligence— divine mind—that is beckoning us to notice and understand its presence.

Kundalini

This is the journey of *Kundalini,* the mythical serpent goddess who rises from base to crown, piercing and awakening each chakra in turn. Kundalini, whose full name is Kundalini-Shakti, is pure energy, guided by intelligence, moving through matter, toward her infinitely beloved partner, Shiva, pure consciousness. Shiva brings intelligence to Shakti's energy, creating everything that exists. When they are joined together, the charge makes a complete circuit. Heaven and earth are united; mind and body are one. This is the true meaning of yoga as union. This is what it means to be whole.

Kundalini is a supercharged, intense concentration of energy that shoots up the spine and pushes through the blockages in the chakras. In Sanskrit, the ancient language of India, these blocks are called *granthis,* which means *knots.* And, of course, in all my workshops, I say the knots in the chakras represent where we *are not,* where we *do not,* where we *will not,* where we *have not,* and where we *cannot.* That's where we're saying: "I'm *not* going to feel that. I'm *not* going to have that." But even the knots are just compressed charge, longing to be free. Kundalini is the concentrated force that can burn through the knots. When we allow those knots to loosen, the Divine can flow through us.

It's the free-flowing expansion of charge that is the essence of the spiritual experience. But it's not free and random; it's free and intelligent. It's not bound, but it does have order. Spirituality is a set of practices to help us come to that experience of divine force flowing through us. But limitlessness, while it is the end of the spectrum that frees up the charge, can also be a place where we get lost. Unbound, it eventually disperses, which is why it's so difficult to sustain these enlightened states.

So we can't help but draw divine essence back *down* into our form as an individual, binding it into new patterns that create our personalities, our behaviors, and our emotions—the patterns that make us human. We are simultaneously humans having a spiritual experience and spiritual beings having a human experience, constantly going back and forth between the finite and the infinite, the mortal and the divine.

Once again, each of us is a storage battery for charge, for the Divine, for the infinite dance between matter and spirit. As the physicist Neil deGrasse Tyson says, "Not only do we live among the stars, but the stars live within us."

In terms of the chakras, the upward current moving from base to crown is the liberating current. That's where we go to liberate ourselves, to find freedom. The downward current is the manifesting current. That's where we create ideas from divine guidance and bring them into form. To reach the Divine and then manifest that Divine as heaven on earth, we need both currents to be open.

What About Beliefs?

The seventh chakra, ultimately representing pure awareness, spends most of its time dwelling in the world of thoughts. These thoughts are busy creating meaning out of what we experience. Your mind right now is making meaning out of these shapes on the paper or screen. It makes them into letters and words that have meaning and lumps the words into sentences, concepts, and ideas.

From the time we are born, we have been making meaning out of our experiences. We interpret Mommy's smiles or frowns to mean that we are good or bad, safe or in danger. Each time Dad gets angry, we make it mean something about what we did, who we are, or how the world is. Each time we're rejected or successful, happy or sad, we add the meaning we make to our internal database about how things are, creating our worldview.

Over time, all those bits of meaning add up to become *beliefs*. Whenever a parent is unavailable or angry, the child might feel distrust or fear. But when something happens repeatedly, like a parent whose punishment is cruel, the meaning we take from each experience begins to add up in our psyche and become beliefs, such as: "I'm not safe." "Life is hard." "I'm not good enough." "There's something wrong with me."

We have an infinite number of beliefs programmed into our awareness. Some of them are consciously chosen, like believing that it's wrong to kill or steal or that eating a certain way is good for you. Some of our beliefs are indoctrinated, such as the religious or cultural beliefs of our parents and friends. But most of our beliefs are running below the radar of awareness. They influence everything we do, but we might not even know there's a hidden belief in there.

Sometimes, beliefs are very subtle. I realized once that I believed I could have anything I wanted as long as I didn't really want it very badly. Therefore, if something was important to me, my unconscious belief was that I could not have it. That was a good belief to change, as it was making me always settle for less than I really wanted.

Meaning and beliefs have a lot of charge, fueling emotion more than logic. The power of beliefs can lead one to throw acid in a girl's face just for going to school, blow themselves up as a suicide bomber, or vote against their best interests. Whether they're religious, political, or personal beliefs, we become quite attached to them—and that attachment is made of charge.

Let's take a common example: a monogamous relationship. If your partner comes home late and you believe he or she is having an affair, you might have a lot of charge about that. If you found out that your partner was just working late, or caught in a traffic jam, or buying you a present on the way home, you'd have a very different experience, even though the reality—your partner not being home for dinner—is the same.

We get especially charged when our beliefs conflict with reality. If we believe we deserve to be paid for work done and someone doesn't pay us, we would understandably have a charge about that. Once we got paid, the charge would diminish. If we believe we should be in a certain kind of relationship, make a certain amount of money, have a perfect body, or even that the world should be a certain way, then we have charge around the places where our reality doesn't match our beliefs—which is most of the time. The mind likes to keep things coherent. It gets fixated when there is cognitive dissonance, often to the point of distraction. I have found that whenever clients are obsessed about something, there is always a contradiction between belief and reality.

Our beliefs tell us how to operate. If I believe that practicing yoga is good for me, then I take myself to a yoga class. If I believe it is right to eat a certain way, or that this is the way to get ahead, get loved, treat others, or have what I want, then that's how I operate in a situation; it's how I behave.

You can think of beliefs as the operating system of your bio-computer. We have mentioned that the body is the hardware, the mind contains the software, and the charge is like the electricity running through the system that allows the hardware and software to connect. But every computer comes with an operating system that interprets the commands, handles the programs, and allows you to write your e-mails. We can't function without beliefs.

While beliefs are the operating system that tells us how to behave and what to do, they also focus consciousness. I focus my attention on whatever I believe is important to me. The podcasts I download, the websites I frequent, the things I choose to do, are all guided by my beliefs of what is important.

But beliefs are not the same as consciousness, which simply makes use of them. Consciousness is something beyond our programs or operating system. In this analogy, consciousness is the "user." It looks at what is happening on the screen and says, "This program isn't what I want. I'll do this instead." Consciousness is the "operator" that has the ability to change the program.

Lion Goodman, co-author of my book *Creating on Purpose,* has made a systematic study of beliefs and how they operate in the human psyche. He tells us that we can consciously examine our beliefs, question whether they are serving us or hindering us, and change them accordingly. When we do, our consciousness is redirected, and as a result, so is our experience. From our new experience, we make new meanings and can reinforce more positive beliefs.

If you have difficulty handling the charge of a situation, it is important to ask yourself what kind of belief is behind your charge. Is that belief serving you? Is it one that you chose consciously or one that was given to you? And even more, is your belief actually true? To more adequately deal with all these questions is more than the scope of this book, but I direct you to Lion Goodman's website, www.ClearYourBeliefs.com.

Our beliefs fixate our charge, keeping it bound, just as we bind charge into the muscles and tissues of the body. The point is not to get rid of the charge but to keep the charge and change the belief.

part iv

CHARGE
and
CHARACTER STRUCTURE

the
CHALLENGES
of
GROWING UP

||||||||||||||||||||||||||||||||||||||||||||||||||||||||||||||||||||||||||||||||||||||

How Character Structure Is Formed

*Blocks are stagnated pools of vital substance
that accumulate in the defensive perimeter and
armor it in dysfunctional patterns that
Reich named character structures.*

JOHN PIERRAKOS

We have now come to a basic understanding of how charge works in the subtle body through the chakra system. But what effect does all this have on the physical body, on our personality, and our life? As it turns out, quite a lot.

At its most basic level, the body *runs on charge*. Without some kind of energy running through us, we wouldn't get up in the morning; we couldn't move or do anything. Everything the body does, from eating to sleeping, from working to exercising, requires energy. The more freely energy runs through the body, the easier it is to do all of these things.

Second, the body *generates* energy for the charge, through breathing air and digesting food. Additionally, we may generate charge by creating crisis, feeling important, or absorbing charge through our relationships.

Third, the body is a *storage battery* for charge. As we've mentioned, larger bodies can better contain excitement, emotions, and stress, while thinner bodies excite more easily yet don't have the means to contain it.

And finally the body is *shaped* by the way charge is held or released in different areas of our physiology—from muscles, tendons, and fat, to organs, glands, and circulatory, digestive, or respiratory systems, including the nervous system itself. Most important, *charge shapes the body while we're growing up*—literally *forming* our body—as we deal with the various tasks and challenges of different stages of childhood. If contraction is part of what we had to do with our charge, the body will become chronically contracted. If pulling our charge up into the head and shoulders is a deeply ingrained habit from childhood, it will actually show up in the body structure as broad shoulders and a commanding head. If blocking our charge in the middle of our belly is what we had to do, the body will thicken in the midsection, and metabolism may be affected. The body shapes itself around the way it holds charge.

The term *character structure* refers to a complex of patterns within the body, mind, and psyche, based on observable physical characteristics, such as body shape, muscle tone, and weight distribution, as well as typical behavior patterns, beliefs, and defenses. Learning about these structures provides a valuable key to understanding yourself and your relationships, as well as your clients, customers, students, children, and friends. By recognizing these complexes and naming them, you have an opportunity to move beyond them, into your true essence. You can also better understand those around you, hold them with more compassion, and learn valuable ways of interacting that support their true self rather than their patterns.

Character structure results from wounding that occurs at specific stages of childhood, where a child fails to get what he needs, is overwhelmed by circumstances, or is otherwise thwarted in the development of important skills. Like all complexes, each structure is a fusion of physical characteristics, emotions, beliefs, behaviors, and personality traits, based on memories, experiences, and imprints from the past. These complexes tend to last a lifetime, unless they are consciously dealt with. They can interfere with our sense of safety, our well-being, the ability to carry on healthy relationships, and general success in life.

These five basic patterns were first identified by Wilhelm Reich, a contemporary of Freud, in the 1930s. Like Freud, Reich practiced psychoanalysis but worked more closely with the body and its energy. He noticed his clients' styles of defensive resistance, which correlated to both patterns of muscular contraction, and further to wounds uncovered through a patient's history. Like geological layers of the earth that pertain to various eras in history, he saw layers of armoring in the body and psyche that related to childhood stages of development.

I have worked with clients' and students' character structures for most of my career and found it to be incredibly useful in terms of diagnosis and treatment. Many other writers have worked with this system, including Alexander Lowen, John Pierrakos, Barbara Brennan, Stephen M. Johnson, Steven Kessler, and me, where I correlated them to the chakras in *Eastern Body, Western Mind*. But the discussion here will focus largely on how each structure deals with and manages their charge.

How the Structures Are Formed

The defensive strategy a child uses to face the challenges of life is dependent upon what skills they have under their belt. A younger child, whose charge is less regulated, has fewer skills to deal with insult than an older child. Infants, for example, have no verbal skills to defend themselves and no ability to fight or run away. If they don't like what's going on, they can cry, which may or may not fix the problem. If it doesn't, their best defense is to tighten their muscles and contract into their core in self-protection. An older child may have verbal skills and a greater sense of self, so she can defend herself with a more skillful command of her charge, using different strategies.

It also depends on what works. If going up into your head and trying to figure everything out makes sense, then the child distances from her body. If latching on to another brings the connection wanted, then the child becomes highly oriented to others. If holding back tears or anger is what works to get one's needs met or avoid trouble, this becomes an unconscious habit. If following the rules offsets rejection or pretending to be powerful works to avoid manipulation, then that becomes part of the behavior. Over time, these strategies become a permanent part of a person's "character armor," defense mechanisms that are hardwired into the body and energy system.

But character structure is determined by additional factors: not only the age of wounding and the skill level available but the type of wounding, the structure of the body, and the amount of charge available to a child at the time. The child who grows up in a volatile family with lots of siblings and intense emotions flying around will likely carry a higher charge than an only child who is left alone and neglected. Of course, like any system, it is not always so cut-and-dried. We may have multiple woundings at different ages. We may exhibit more than one layer of character armor and a variety of defenses and beliefs. Most of us do.

What is important to remember is that these structures are *patterns* that are lodged into the body, *patterns that are held in place by charge.* And these patterns have a cost. They limit the full and free expression of who we are. Their dysfunction ranges from mild to extreme as they limit our freedom, authenticity, and ability to form intimate relationships. Learning to recognize these patterns gives us the choice to distance from them, disable them, and eventually move out of them completely into greater presence of our essential being.

The next five chapters will look at each of these structures in detail. To get an overview of how all the structures play out in different aspects of our lives, take a look at the chart on pages 212–213, which correlates each pattern by age of wounding, beliefs, defense strategies, and other characteristics.

If you would like to do a general assessment of yourself, make check marks next to the listings that feel true for you, even making two or three check marks for aspects that are more strongly true. You may fit many things in a single structure or fit some traits to a T, while other traits, not at all. Like any personality system, not everyone fits neatly into pigeonholes, but the chart can give you a general idea of how these complexes work together. As we heal and move along our path, we may have grown out of some of these defenses. We realize we used to be like this or that but no longer use those strategies. On the other hand, when we work through one layer of defense, we might uncover another one underneath.

Notice the columns that have the most check marks. That is probably your dominant pattern. But since we rarely have just one pattern, you will probably have check marks in other columns as well that indicate tendencies in your personality but not your primary default pattern. When you read about each structure more deeply, you might notice your charge coming up in the patterns that are most relevant to you.

It's important to avoid looking at this as some kind of pathology or yet another system that tells you what's wrong with you. Rather, these are characterological patterns that can lead to deeper awareness. If you can recognize that you use those patterns and become more cognizant of why and how, you have a better chance of getting out of them. If you can recognize these patterns in your partners, children, friends, or co-workers, you can avoid the pitfalls of getting hooked by their behavior, hold them in more compassion, and become more skillful at dealing with their personalities.

The result is a greater ability to live in one's true essence and free flow of charge. We can be *in charge* of our patterns, instead of our patterns running our charge. In the following chapters, we will look at each structure in depth.

The Five Basic Character Structures

Classical Names	Schizoid	Oral	Masochist	Psychopath	Rigid
Alternate Names	Creative, Leaving, Unwanted Child	Lover, Merging, Under-nourished Child	Endurer, Defeated Child, Overman-aged Child	Challenger-Defender, Aggressive, Betrayed Child	Achiever, Perfection-ist, Hurried Child
Age of Wounding	Utero to 6 months	6 months to 2 years	18 months to 3 years	2.5 to 4 years	3.5 to 5 years
Parent	Angry, fright-ened, dis-embodied	Depriv-ing, over-whelmed	Intrusive, enmeshed, controlling	Seductive or authori-tarian	Sexually rejecting, cold, rule follower
Charge and Holding Pattern	Holds together, high charge, jumpy	Holds on, collapsed, low charge	Holds in, dense, blocked charge	Holds up, outwardly directed, high charge	Holds back, surface, high charge
Gifts	Con-nected to spirit, in-telligent, creative	Loving, generous, caring, flowing	Loyal, steady, patient	Strong will, big energy, charis-matic	Accom-plished, optimistic, structured
Challenges	Embodi-ment	Receiv-ing, self-reliance	Individua-tion, tak-ing action	Vulnerabil-ity, trust, yielding	Feeling authentic self, owning shadow

Classical Names	Schizoid	Oral	Masochist	Psychopath	Rigid
Fear	Falling apart, going crazy	Abandonment	Exposure, humiliation	Surrender to others	Surrender to feelings
Doubts	Right to exist	Right to have	Right to act	Right to love	Right to want
Illusion	My mind is my body	Love will solve everything	I'm trying to please you	It's all a matter of will	Performance is everything
Central Emotion	Fear	Sadness	Resentment, guilt	Anger	Shame
Personality	Mental, creative, scattered	Needy, dependent, merging	Heavy, withdrawn, feels stuck	Power hungry, obstinate, contrary	Proud, competitive, motivated
Defense Strategy	Withdraw, escape	Fixate on others, collapse	Resist, hide	Dominate, control	Compete, perform, follow rules
Eyes	Vacant, scattered	Pleading	Suffering, confused	Commanding	Sparkling, bright
Body Signs	Thin, wiry, angular	Round, soft, sunken chest	Compressed, thick, dense	Broad shoulders, loose pelvis, strong head	Attractive, tight, well toned, fit
Healing	Grounding, embodiment	Find core, stand on own two feet	Move resistance to action, say "No"	Trust something bigger than you are	Acknowledge needs, feelings, shadow

chapter 19

the
SCHIZOID
STRUCTURE

||||||||||||||||||||||||||||||||||||||||||||||||||||||||||||||||||||||||||||||||

Caught Between the Worlds

When Serena first walked into my workshop, I was struck by her attractively chiseled features, bright eyes, and tall, thin body. Hers was a delicate beauty, reminiscent of a china doll. It almost seemed she would break and shatter, were she not handled carefully.

She smiled and shook my hand but energetically drew back ever so slightly when I met her gaze. I sensed her shyness and the intensity of charge in her delicate body. After scanning the half-filled room for a seat, she finally chose one at the back and carefully sat down, wrapping her shawl around her.

As the workshop progressed, she seemed attentive, taking copious notes. When we talked about the first chakra, she became quieter and more withdrawn, almost pale. I could tell something was triggering her, so I was surprised when I asked for a volunteer for the grounding exercise and she raised her hand. Getting up in front of a room full of strangers to expose your vulnerability isn't easy for anyone. But early on in a workshop, before people really know one another, it's even more frightening. Recognizing her as a Schizoid character structure whose main issue is *fear,* I knew this was a very courageous act.

I encouraged her to push down into her legs, energetically pressing her feet down and out, bending and straightening her knees. It was clear that opening the channels in her legs was a complete mystery to her. She was doing her best to follow the mechanics of my instructions, but she could not push energy *through* her legs. It was as if she found her feet by going around the outside, moving them like a puppet master moves a puppet, rather than feeling the energy from within.

Very quickly, however, her whole body started to tremble with charge. Knowing that her first chakra ability to ground that charge was still weak, I didn't want her to get overcharged, so I had her gently push against my hands as a way to discharge, while grounding and saying the words, "I am in here." At first the words were mechanical, almost a question, but after she repeated the phrase a few more times, the truth of that statement started to take hold and a new solidity came into her body. She had the sense, perhaps for the first time, of truly occupying her body. She looked brighter and more alive as she walked back to her seat, still a bit shaky, but with the sense that something she couldn't quite define was taking place within her.

Serena was a classic example of the Schizoid character structure, also called the Creative, the Leaving Pattern, and the Unwanted Child. Not that the child necessarily *was* unwanted, but their experience was of *feeling* unwanted, out of place, or not belonging.

The Schizoid Source of Wounding

Imagine, if you will, that you were suddenly struck by a terrible illness that took away your physical coordination, wiped out your entire memory, including the ability to speak or understand language, and dropped you soaking wet and stark naked onto a foreign planet. Nothing at all is familiar. There are creatures you've never seen before and sounds you cannot interpret. You can't seem to operate your body very well.

Sounds horrifying, doesn't it? As you imagine this scenario, notice what your body does energetically. Does it tense up, drawing into its core? Pull upward, away from the ground? Rush up into the head? Do you find yourself holding your breath?

Now imagine that a loving figure, larger than life, gently and tenderly picks you up, wraps you in a blanket, and brings you to a warm breast, making soft cooing sounds. You feel safe. You could now let go of holding so tightly on to yourself. You could relax and begin to look around. *You could arrive.*

This is the condition of our birth, as we finally emerge from the many hours of contractions, bashing our head against the opening of the womb, at last to be pushed out into the cold and unfamiliar physical world. No matter how we were born, the contrast between the womb and the outer world is stark. But how we came through our birth has a lot to do with how comfortably we engage with our own bodies and the world around us.

If we were welcomed and protected, held firmly, and grounded into this reality with love and warmth, we have a good chance of sensing that we will survive. The nervous system can relax and allow itself to begin processing this strange new experience of having a body.

But what if there was no one to hold you and calm you, no warm body to regulate your nervous system and communicate that everything is going to be okay? What if you were whisked off to a nursery, pulled away from the only flesh that is familiar, placed alone under bright lights, in the vicinity of numerous other traumatized and screaming babies? You would feel a sense that something was terribly wrong, something your nervous system cannot understand or adapt to. Unable to speak or move your limbs effectively, there is only one thing you could do to defend yourself: *contract.*

If the situation isn't remedied, you might stay in that contracted state, muscularly drawing into your core, imprinted by fear at the primary core of your being. Just like squeezing a tube of toothpaste pushes a substance out the top of the tube, this contraction pushes the prodigious charge of the life force upward, into the head and even outside the body.

This stimulates the upper chakras prematurely, as the mental apparatus has no way of making sense of anything it experiences. There is no context for what is going on; you can't understand the language, you don't recognize your surroundings, you don't know how to make anything happen. Listen and look as you might, it would not yield any understanding. But that wouldn't stop you from trying.

Instead, your upper chakras would open out of sequence; impressions would pour into your consciousness, with nothing to ground them. If you are not touched and held, "living in your head" can become a permanent state, ever present as you build your body through childhood, as you engage with new things in adulthood, and as you continually try to manage the charge of terror that is now hardwired into your body and running your unconscious mind. The result is a very capable intellect living in a contracted body that has very little insulation between the inner and outer worlds.

And no wonder. Such a terrifying experience would make you long for the peace of the womb you occupied for the last nine months, or perhaps for the spirit world, floating free without a body. That would be home to you, not this tiny body, unprotected in a strange and dangerous world.

The Schizoid/Creative character structure has the youngest wounding of any of the five major structures. It might even occur in the womb, if the mother is ambivalent about her pregnancy, resistant to having a child, or even if the mother is Schizoid herself. This may create an energetic contraction throughout the mother's body, which communicates to the child on an unconscious, sensory level: "There's not enough room for me. I am unwanted. I am not safe. I might die." This is not a cognitive thought, as the brain is not yet developed enough for that; *it's a cellular imprint of helplessness in the face of danger.* If it is mildly charged, it can be a source of fear or discomfort. If it is highly charged, it feels like terror.

This wounding can also occur as a result of birth trauma or any difficulties arising during the first six months of life. This is when an infant's life force goes into forming a body and learning about the conditions of the physical world: eating, digesting, and dealing with edges, boundaries, and gravity. If the child fails to bond well with the mother, is separated from her, finds the mother angry or toxic, or is born into an environment of danger, the young infant, who has no verbal or muscular skills, can only draw inward, deep into herself, as a protection. This can produce a lifetime of energetic and bodily contraction, if it is not remedied.

In terms of chakras, this creates a deficiency in the first chakra and an excess in the upper chakras. Embodiment doesn't fully take place and is sometimes accompanied by a strong desire *not* to be here, even keeping the body small and thin. Such a person has one foot in the physical world and another in the spiritual world.

The only place to expand is into the mental or spiritual worlds, places that transcend the boundaries of the physical world and allow welcome relief from the constant constriction. Perhaps the child is trying to return to the etheric world they just came from, with only one foot in the waters of this world, never coming into full embodiment, often unsure of whether they even want to be here. Instead the intellect and fantasy offer a welcome antidote to reality, an expansive sense of home and safety that they can't find in this world.

Without the remedy of safety and assurance from loving caretakers, a child builds her body around this energetic contraction. Rather than expanding *into* the world and taking up space, the child is instead shrinking *from* the world, keeping herself small. Contraction is equated to survival, and letting go of it feels like a matter of life and death. It's a wicked double bind: holding on to all this charge is terribly uncomfortable, but letting go of it feels like losing the only sense of identity you have.

Such contraction is not merely in the body. It may include contracting from relationships, careers, or any challenging situations. It can make the voice suddenly get small and childlike when charge arises in the body. It can make fearful eyes, and I have even seen a high degree of scoliosis (misalignment of the spine) as if the child were trying to turn away from something that felt hostile, deep in the core of their being.

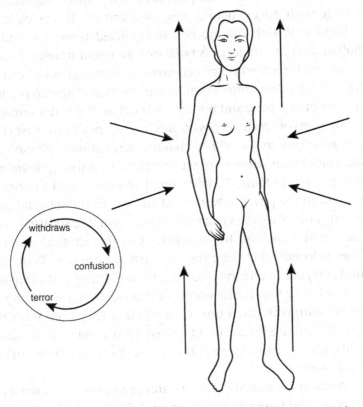

Figure 10 Schizoid Character Structure: Thin, contracted, drawn upward

Charge Pattern

If the body is muscularly and energetically contracted into the core, it tends to be tall and thin, or sometimes just petite. It's as if the person is afraid to take up space and may even question their right to be here. Consider the way a river creates a faster and more turbulent flow when it passes through a narrow channel, or the way constricted blood vessels lead to high blood pressure. In the same way, when the body is contracted, the charge moves through a narrower opening and becomes more intense. Without a wider and more solid core channel through which to move the energy, a person charges up very quickly, but even a little charge can feel overwhelming.

Because the thin body of the Schizoid doesn't have a lot of shielding between the inside and outside worlds, things tend to impact them more strongly than they might others. Loud noises, harsh words, bright lights, or intense situations—both positive (such as a party with numerous people) and negative (such as a threatening situation)—can feel like too much. This makes for a highly sensitive person whose most basic defense is to energetically withdraw from the situation.

Overwhelm is the inability to deal effectively with the challenges at hand. While all the character structures result from feelings of overwhelm, they occur in different ways, so the response is different for each structure. In the Schizoid, any kind of overwhelm stimulates the original contraction. Steven Kessler, in his book *The 5 Personality Patterns*,[1] calls this the *Leaving Pattern*, because to another person, it feels like they are withdrawing from the situation at hand. They might walk out on an argument; they might space out during sex; or they might have to leave the party and go outside where it's quiet. They can also energetically leave, even though physically they might still be present. There is a kind of vacancy or spaciness that feels like the person just isn't all there.

If withdrawal can't take place, then the Schizoid fragments their charge. What does fragmentation look like? A person might rapidly change subjects, exhibit jumpy or erratic movements, scatter their attention in many directions, or, in more pathological cases, it can even show up as multiple personalities, each of whom carries a piece of the core charge. Some people fragment their charge through having several jobs or multiple lovers, moving from place to place or simply having too many interests in different things. Such a person might say, "I feel like I'm all over the place." And indeed they are.

The root of the word *Schizoid* means *split*, and there's a way this structure splits from their charge. This does not imply schizophrenic, by the way, which is a far more serious condition. Rather, it simply means that awareness splits off from the body, and even from aspects of their own self, such as sexuality, emotions, power, or love. (Notice these are associations with the lower chakras.) One of my students with this structure remarked after a workshop, "I now realize that I have spent my whole life watching myself from a distance, as if I were watching someone else in a movie."

Many Schizoids are highly spiritual people, often drawn to yoga and meditation, fasting, ascension philosophies, or intellectual realms. Practicing yoga may help them find their bodies, but in some cases the pursuit of transcendence can be used as a form of escape and exacerbate the defense. Meditation comes naturally to them, and even though they are thin, they often have an easy time fasting or removing themselves from the rigors of daily life. They have a large propensity for being alone and have learned to come back into balance when they are by themselves, away from others. Naturally, they tend toward introversion.

Recognize the Pattern When:

- You feel an urgent need to retreat.
- You live in your head and deny your body.
- You feel scared even though there is no current threat.
- You are scattering or fragmenting your energy.
- You feel alone and isolated.
- You use spirituality as an escape.

Gifts of the Schizoid Pattern

Like all the structures, there are gifts that are developed, gifts that can be kept, even when one works through their patterns and moves beyond the structure. In the Schizoid, these gifts have to do with connection to spirit, intelligence, and creativity. The following is a description of the gifts in more detail.

Mental agility. Because of their high sensitivity, this structure tends to be intellectually, spiritually, and creatively gifted. When not triggered by circumstance, they have the ability to think things through, to see multiple perspectives. Their intellectual gifts draw them toward professions such as computer programming, scholarship and research, academic teaching, or other realms that deal with abstract ideas.

Access to other planes. Since Schizoid types are not fully in the mundane world, they have the ability to reach into the spirit world. They receive guidance from beyond, see angels or channel entities, and sense past lives. To people who are more practical and grounded, this can seem naïve or silly, yet to the Schizoid pattern, this connection to the unseen world is very real. They are highly intuitive, introspective, and spiritually oriented, in the classic sense of the word.

Creativity. This is also called the Creative structure, as it is often found in artists, writers, musicians, or poets. They easily come up with creative solutions to problems and are quite able to think outside of the box (having never fit in the box to begin with!). But even if their artistry is excellent, as it often is, they have a hard time getting their work recognized, since being in the limelight can trigger the fear complex. They are often the undiscovered geniuses whose gifts go unacknowledged.

Light living. Schizoid types are usually happy with fewer possessions and like to remain fluid and light. Since they aren't strongly connected to the earth anyway, people, places, and things don't have a lot of hold on them. They often move their domicile frequently, and are averse to accumulation. Money isn't a big pull, but if they have some wealth, it is sealed up in a bank somewhere, while their spending is quite frugal. I knew one man who had *millions* in the bank but fretted over the cost of a cheap bottle of wine for a potluck.

Humility. Schizoids tend not to have big egos and instead prefer to be in service, choosing jobs where they can work quietly on their own, in relative peace and freedom. They give wonderful support to others and are great at thinking ahead.

Healing the Schizoid

I once had a client who was an attractive woman in her early 40s. She came to me, ostensibly, because she had never had a second date. When I asked her why, she told me that she gets so excited and nervous that her throat closes up and she becomes unable to speak. I could understand that sitting there for a whole evening, unable to make conversation, certainly didn't bode well for a second date. I asked her if she felt scared on the date, and she replied that she was more excited than scared but that the excitement felt like fear to her body and made her contract. This was beyond her conscious control.

We worked together to reframe the pattern in terms of charge. I taught her to befriend her charge, seeing it as part of her aliveness, and how to track charge in her body. Instead of helplessly letting the charge get stuck in her throat chakra, I taught her to push it down into her feet—to give the charge a place to go that was solid. I don't know the long-term outcome of her love life, but having a place to put her charge helped her tremendously in just a few sessions.

The Schizoid's primary concern is safety. They can't heal without it. But safety can't always be supplied by the outside world—there is no guarantee that anything is completely safe. It must be provided through opening the channels in the legs and learning how to ground.

When safety is not established, it's hard for the nervous system to relax. This moves beyond one's conscious control and becomes hardwired into the nervous system and charge pattern. In other words, you might know that the door is locked, yet be unable to let go of your hypervigilance and feel at ease. Therefore, almost any situation that brings up any kind of charge simultaneously brings up fear, which then becomes a habit of the body.

For an infant, safety comes from being held, rocked, bounced, and appropriately touched by loving parents. In order to heal the split from the body, the Schizoid needs physical touch and lots of it, but it's not something they typically seek. Physical activity, regular massage, even deep-tissue bodywork (as long as it's not too painful) are absolutely essential. However, this type is more likely to seek purely talk therapy, even choosing a therapist who works through Skype or phone, rather than in person.

If you are a therapist for whom touch is inappropriate for your scope of practice, it is essential to assign your Schizoid-patterned client regular massages or other forms of touch and physical activity. It is also essential to have something solid to push against to run charge through your body. This can be the floor, as in the basic grounding exercise, or it can be a wall. If you can use physical contact, it can be helpful to have the person press into your hands while connecting through the eyes.

It's also important to continually refer to the body. While talking about any kind of issue or feeling, or if you see any kind of charge arise, ask, "Where do you feel that in your body?" This helps bridge the mind-body gap and starts to form an important relationship with the inner processes of the body.

Ultimately, Schizoids need to learn how to manage their charge by harvesting it into the tissues. Yet they can only do so when their body expands, giving them more room to contain the charge. Until then, simple discharging can help them become more comfortable.

Schizoid Expansion Exercise

The following exercise can create remarkable shifts in the Schizoid's disembodiment and help them become more present and grounded. It helps to counteract the chronic contraction into the core, by producing a feeling of expansion that allows them to drop down inside themselves and into their body.

I ask the person to stand in front of me and explain that with their permission, I am going to press on various parts of the body with one of my hands. Whenever I touch them, I ask them to take a deep breath, and then on the exhalation, to push that part of their body against my hand.

I begin in the extremities, often with the upper arms. First one side then the other, I instruct the person not to lean against my hand but to push out from their core and imagine widening the energetic space they live in. As they push against me, I offer a slight amount of resistance—enough to make them use real effort but not so much that they can't move outward.

I then go to the thighs, hips, shoulders, upper and lower back. Needless to say, I avoid the buttocks, breasts, or anything near the genital area.

As I gradually work my way from periphery to core, my final steps are to push against their third chakra, then the sternum. The very final step is to have the person draw their hands up, palms facing outward, close to their body, and then push into the resistance of my hands as they straighten their arms, pushing me away. This final step teaches them that rather than going away themselves, they can make something in their environment go away. This allows them to take up more room, instead of shrinking away from what they don't like.

The result is that the person feels larger and simultaneously more grounded and more grown-up. With the expansion at the core, there is room for the spirit to drop down into the body.

the
ORAL
STRUCTURE

||||||||||||||||||||||||||||||||||||||||||||||||||||||||||||||||||||||||||||

The Empathic Lover

Sandra smiled warmly with a gentle presence that was immediately relaxing. Her round body and soft features had a sweetness that was simultaneously childlike and motherly. Though she behaved as anyone would on meeting someone for the first time, her energetic body rushed ahead of her physical body, as if to merge with mine.

When she sat down, I noticed her shoulders were rounded, her chest somewhat concave, and her initially friendly eyes held a veiled sadness. Even though we were just beginning our session, she seemed ready to cry at any moment.

When I asked why she had come to me, she immediately began talking about her husband. Everything she said was about her partner, and very little about herself. I asked her what her own needs were, and she replied about how she needed her partner to be different, still focusing outside herself.

It might seem paradoxical, but Sandra was very emotional, yet she didn't feel her own core very well, jumping over her own inner cues. She often felt overwhelmed by the needs of others—as she could feel their needs more than she could feel her own. She was highly oriented toward her relationships, her children, and her social life. She told me that she felt slightly depressed when she spent time alone, but came to life when she was serving others, which gave her a sense of purpose.

Sandra is an example of an Oral character structure, also called the Lover, the Need Structure, the Merging Pattern, and the Undernourished Child.

The Oral Source of Wounding

During the first six months of life (the Schizoid wounding stage), an infant's attention and energy is largely focused on the struggle to operate the body and deal with the physical world, in short to survive. Once eating, digesting, and getting used to the environment have taken place, a child then becomes more aware of her caretakers.

Learning that these big people you see every day are the ones who feed you, hold you, and care for you has hopefully built a level of trust and security and limbic resonance. With an embodied sense that you will survive, the emotional needs now surface, highlighting your relationship with others.

This is a time when the child is still too young to supply any of her own needs. She does not yet have verbal language, and her world is made of sensory impressions that stimulate, soothe, or direct her charge. Naturally, much of that charge is focused outside herself, toward the people who feed and care for her.

The child's needs are expressed *unconsciously* through emotion. I say unconsciously because the child is not actively sensing her needs but rather *reactively* sensing them. In other words, the child doesn't think, "This milk is too hot," or, "Something is pinching me"; it's just an immediate movement of charge through the body that expresses itself to anyone around. It generally comes out through the mouth in wails and through the limbs in movement. In a healthy family environment, the child's crying gets her fed, her diapers changed, or her nervous system regulated when she's upset.

Crying or laughing, smiling or frowning, looking scared or angry—these are the emanations moving through this small body from within to without. They are not filtered, analyzed, or even cognitive. Their purpose is to connect the child's interior experience with someone who responds and can mediate things to enhance pleasure and reduce pain.

At this stage, charge simply comes in and goes out, without inhibition on the part of the child. Charge comes into the body through nourishment and nurturance—*food, touch, love,* and *attention.* If the child is undernourished in any of these essential areas, the body remains chronically *undercharged.* The child doesn't get to feel full or satisfied. As a result, consciousness fixates outside the self, always looking to see where she might get her needs met. She becomes hyperaware of the moods and emotions of her caretakers, at the cost of feeling herself. As the awareness shifts outward, it shifts away from the interior core, causing further depletion.

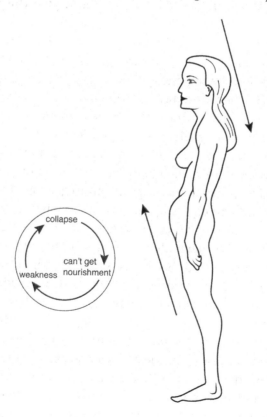

Figure 11 Oral Character Structure: Collapsed chest, passive ground

Charge Pattern

This sense of depletion, deprivation, and "not having enough" can then become a persistent framework for interacting with the outside world. A body with too little charge doesn't have the energy for self-assertion or to take on challenges.

Where the Schizoid pattern is to withdraw, the Oral pattern tends to *merge* with others. Always seeking nourishment from outside, relationships are seen as a source from which to feed. Oral characters love to love! They fall in love easily, often with no reservation, only to find that their lover doesn't fulfill their needs as well as they hoped. When this happens, they try to give even more, becoming the caretakers they wished they'd had. When their giving doesn't produce the result of getting their needs met, they can feel resentful. "After all I've given you, this is all I get in return?"

Most of this is completely unconscious. It happens below the radar of awareness. On the surface, people with the Oral pattern are generous and loving and genuinely try to do good for others. The trouble is, they get drained in the process, not having enough charge to begin with, and then deplete themselves further by giving even more of their precious charge to others. As much as the oral pattern needs to receive, the defense paradoxically blocks that reception, with difficulty receiving love from others even when it is given, with digestive problems in getting nutrients from their food and with challenges in asking for what they want.

In relationships, Orals can be overly attached and clingy, even meddlesome and co-dependent. They are highly sensitive to rejection or deprivation, and their greatest fear is abandonment. Their defense is to *hold on*: to others, to the past, to grudges, beliefs, and behaviors. When you don't have enough, it's hard to let go of what you do have. Often they stay in undernourishing relationships longer than they should, preferring to get less than what they want rather than face the challenge of their aloneness.

The past deprivation often creates a countermovement of *indulgence,* and people with the Oral pattern, fixated at the oral stage of development, when nourishment comes in largely through the mouth, may overindulge through eating, talking, smoking, drinking, and sex. For this reason, Orals are sometimes called the Lover, as they are giving, merging, and hungry for connection.

Because the body is chronically undercharged, the oral pattern exhibits a bit of a slumping posture, as if everything is collapsing downward. In standing, their knees are often locked, which throws the hips forward, the chest back, and the head forward, bringing all the chakras out of alignment. When the shoulders are rounded forward and the chest concave, the belly pushes outward to compensate. With a collapsed chest, their breath tends to be shallow, which further contributes to less charge. If you think of how your body feels when you're tired, that is the semipermanent state of the Oral-patterned body—relaxed, but not very energized. The muscles tend to remain soft and lack definition; however, they are highly flexible and fluid, preferring movement to stillness.

The need for nourishment and love of eating often creates obesity or weight problems for the Oral pattern. Oral women tend to have large, pendulous breasts, while men may have "man breasts" and a soft, pudgy layer of extra weight. Dieting is difficult for the Oral pattern, as it stimulates the wound of deprivation. You often see diet-and-binge cycles that fail to bring the body into its normal size.

Recognize the Pattern When:

- You feel collapsed and overwhelmed.
- You give your energy away to others.
- You feel needy.
- You hang on too tightly to relationships.
- You overindulge in food, smoking, drinking, or sex.
- You can't maintain your charge when alone.

Gifts of the Oral Pattern

The Orals' gifts are many, and because they are so busy sharing them, it's easy to miss the fact that they are undercharged and needing to receive.

Lovers of life. Oral-patterned people are highly social and enjoy life fully, relishing its richness. They tend to be warm, personable, and openhearted. They make great cooks and love to entertain. They are sensuous and enjoy colors, sounds, tastes, and new experiences.

Generous. This is the type of person you can call anytime, day or night—they will listen to your problems and give you support. They know what it's like to be deprived, so they are highly generous, giving away what little they have in order to benefit others. If they have money, they share the bounty with others. In their work life they tend toward giving professions, such as nurses, teachers, bodyworkers, and therapists, and they are generally good at what they do. They lead with kindness and compassion.

Highly relational. Relationship is the primary focus of Oral types, so they make devoted friends, partners, or parents. They are sensitive to the needs of others, often more so than themselves. They're great social organizers and love bringing people together.

Easygoing. Being somewhat undercharged, Oral types don't anger easily. They tend to be more fluid than fixed and can roll with the punches. They are generally forgiving of others' faults.

Healing the Oral Pattern

In order for the Oral pattern to heal, they need to increase the amount of charge in their body and learn to contain that charge, rather than letting it leak out and dissipate. This requires charging exercises, such as Opening the Leg Channels (page 124), increasing oxygen intake through deeper breathing, and finding their own spiritual source of energy, rather than trying to get it from other people.

At the same time, they need to avoid discharging activities, such as crying, yelling, or talking too much. Orals tend toward dependency, so getting an Oral person to feel her own ground and stand on her own two feet is essential. Physical exercise is important for strengthening the body.

Since Orals are naturally nurturing toward others, they need to turn that nurturing toward themselves and develop healthy self-care. Orals need to identify their needs and take personal responsibility to get them met. Developing boundaries is necessary to keep their own charge and strengthen their core. If they fail to access their own core and assert their boundaries, they can often invade the boundaries of others.

Boundary Exercise

For this exercise, both people are standing some distance apart, 10–15 feet, if possible. (I have been known to go out into a parking lot to create enough space with some clients!)

I tell the person I am working with that we are going to do a boundary exercise and that I am going to slowly walk toward him. I tell him that he is allowed to do whatever comes naturally to him as I walk toward his personal space.

I take one step at a time, carefully observing the level of charge in the body. I watch the eyes, the hand movements, the face, and the breath for any signs of arousal. Often I see these signs before a person takes action to stop my approach, but the first time around, I simply notice and keep quiet. Sometimes a person takes no action whatsoever and allows me to push them backward, sometimes all the way to the wall. (I do this gently, however!) Other times, someone says *stop*, or puts their hands up as a boundary.

This gives me a sense of the person's ability to sense their boundary and to defend it appropriately.

I then point out where I saw the activation arise, stepping back to that distance. I say something like, "I saw you tense up when I was standing here, and I saw you flinch when I stood here, and you visibly drew back when I stood here but never said stop."

Then I repeat the exercise, giving them feedback on these subtle activations as I step forward again. I encourage them to notice these messages from their body and to respond accordingly with words and/or motions, such as putting the hands up.

Once the boundary is established, I can take it to the next step, which is asking him to defend an invasion of his boundary. I push into his hands and ask him to push back against me, using any words that come naturally, such as "Back off," "Stop right there," or "Get away." When these words are said with full charge, I stop and allow the person to feel the exhilaration and charge of having set a clear boundary.

Earth Skiing

If you go waterskiing, you begin down in the water, knees bent. As the boat begins to move forward, you have to keep your feet in front of you to avoid being pulled over onto your face. This exercise uses the same principle, but you are pushing into the floor instead of water.

Two people stand across from each other and join wrist to wrist, right hand to the other's right, left hand to the left. Then each person bends their knees as if sitting in a chair. It is important not to bend so deeply that your hips descend below your knees, but to keep your thighs parallel to the floor.

Each person increases the pressure of their feet against the floor as a resistance to being pulled over. The more one person pushes into the floor, the more the other one has to push as well. Often the thighs will begin to tremble with the effort. That's a sign that charge is moving through the legs.

Once this gets going, try to keep that dynamic connection with the earth as both people slowly pull each other up to standing. Make sure the connection doesn't break. If it does, go back down and try again.

The result is a feeling of being pulled directly into your ground, standing on your own two feet, and energizing the legs.

chapter 21

the
ENDURER
STRUCTURE

||||||||||||||||||||||||||||||||||||||||||||||||||||||||||||||||||||||||||||||||

The Masochist

Christopher wasn't what you would consider overweight, but his body was dense and stocky. Outwardly, he seemed solid as a rock, but it was difficult to feel what was going on inside him. He spoke with a heavy voice, and his body had very little animation, even when talking about difficult things.

As he began to tell me why he was seeking therapy, he said he felt *stuck*—describing a kind of damned-if-you-do-and-damned-if-you-don't scenario. He wasn't really happy in his job as an accountant, but it paid the bills. He felt stuck in his marriage of 17 years, having resigned himself to the relationship being "as good as it gets," which, in his estimation, wasn't very good. He preferred to spend time alone, puttering around his backyard, playing with the dog. He dabbled at a few hobbies, never sticking to anything for long, with a pile of unfinished projects all over the house. He had some buried dreams, but they were quickly squashed by a million excuses as to why they could never happen.

As I slowly gained entry into his personal world, I noticed how critical he was of himself. He obsessed about how he should have chosen a different career, married a different woman, gotten an advanced degree, or that he should be earning more money. He told me that he was lazy and didn't follow through on things.

He'd had a chance to rise to a more managerial level in his work, but he'd sabotaged it at the last minute by not showing up for the interview, and someone else had gotten the job. Listening to him rattle off all this negativity was enough to make me feel a heaviness in my own body.

Christopher looked at his life as a series of obligations, which made his daily outlook seem grim. "I have to take care of my mother, who is alone and aging. I have to help out my sister financially, because she just separated from her husband, so I can't take the vacation I wanted. I have to deal with the kids and don't really get weekends off. I have to get myself together, but just can't seem to make any movement. I have to eat better, drink less, exercise more, but I hate doing those things. And then I get mad at myself for failing."

When he thought about future scenarios, he transferred a similar negativity. "What if I change careers and I'm just as bored? What if I move to a new city and wish I hadn't? What if I leave my wife and can't find something better?" With this kind of thinking, he was defeated before he could start.

He generally perceived life as offering him no choice. In personal relationships, he lived in a cycle of victim and blaming. He was deeply uncomfortable with conflict and would simply appease rather than risk rocking the boat. That left him resentful toward his partner, whom he blamed for always getting her way, even though he rarely made assertions about what he wanted.

Not that Christopher was irresponsible. Far from the case. He was a steady and dependable provider for his family, loyal to a fault, and a kind and considerate person who loved his children deeply. But he lived in a private, silent suffering, resulting from his masochistic tendency to deny himself in order to avoid disappointing someone else.

Does any of this sound familiar?

Then you may exhibit the pattern of the Endurer. Traditionally, it's called the Masochist, because of the tendency to internally criticize, hurt oneself, and, like the Oral pattern, deny one's own needs. But since most people abhor identifying with the word *masochist*, I prefer to call this pattern the "Endurer," because their gift and their curse is that they are able to endure situations better than other types. Because they *can* endure, they do, and this creates suffering and grief—not from big losses or hurts, but from the constant resignation to circumstances that are less than optimal.

The Endurer Source of Wounding

Even under the best of conditions, the terrible twos are a difficult time for parents. I remember my son used to throw his shoes out the second-story window when I was trying to get him dressed in the morning before I went to work, just to exert his will. Two-year-olds thwart authority, act stubbornly, insist on "me" and "mine," and often say *no* just because the parent says *yes.* This is the time when kids throw temper tantrums and generally resist everything they're told to do. Thankfully, this stage eventually passes, and the child learns to accept authority without sacrificing his own self.

This stage (18 months to 3 years) is the early part of the third chakra developmental phase when a child is discovering the power of his will. If autonomy and personal power are thwarted, then we approach life from a preexisting sense of defeat. Without access to our will, we become victims of our circumstances. Without an autonomous self that can differentiate, disagree, or otherwise be assertive, Endurers feel resigned to accept what they are given. Such resignation produces a state of mild depression.

There are many ways that parents can interfere with this important third chakra development. They can be authoritarian, with rules that can't be questioned. They can force the child to endure difficult things, such as abuse from a parent, sibling, or relative. They can punish the child for acts of autonomy or use shame as a means of control.

This creates a conflict in the child between their personal will and the desire to be loved. Unconsciously it becomes an either/or conflict—either he can be true to himself and sacrifice love and approval, or he can give up himself in order to be loved.

Most insidious is the parent (usually the mother) who controls the child through a seeming sweetness. "Oh, my little Charlie would never steal a cookie like that nasty little boy next door, now would he? He's Mommy's favorite and he's always such a good little boy." With such a comment, Charlie is faced with pleasing his mother or being autonomous—and the mother wins.

One young man I worked with had a mother who had expressed her "love" through meticulously choosing everything for him all the way through high school. She chose his clothes, the décor of his room, his playmates, and his activities. But she never hugged him or said, "I love you." It was no wonder that as an adult, this person suffered from chronic fatigue (no energy or will to do anything) and had trouble knowing what he wanted.

It's important for a child (or anyone, for that matter) to have the right to say *no*. It's interesting that parents expect their teenagers to have the ability to "Just say no" to drugs and sex, when many children have been robbed of their "no" all through childhood. My own parents tossed a bucket of ice water on me whenever I threw a temper tantrum, just because they read it in a book somewhere. Just when I was letting out my charge, which was my expression of a "No!" they shocked me out of my anger. Finding my fire and standing my ground has been an issue for me ever since. Maybe that's why I've come to understand charge so well!

The alternate names of this structure reflect various aspects of this wounding. The Masochist, the Autonomy Structure, the Overmanaged Child, the Controlled Child, and the Defeated Child all point to the fact that this child did not get to have his full autonomy as a separate and unique being and, as a result, never fully developed his power and will.

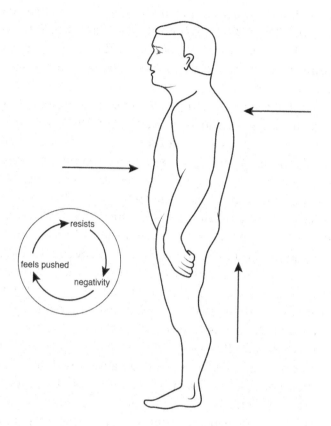

Figure 12 Endurer Character Structure: Dense tissue, holding in the middle

Charge Pattern

If the third chakra represents the element fire, then the Endurer character structure has a smoky, smoldering fire, like burning damp wood. The fire isn't absent; it's just blocked from being outwardly asserted. The fire, which is blocked from action, turns instead against the self, through a vicious inner critic or other self-sabotaging behavior. When the child feels defeated before he even starts, his charge is dampened by a sense of futility.

Think of how you might have felt if you'd been sent to your room, unjustly, during your favorite TV program. You would do as you're told but inwardly resist, a pattern I call *outer compliance and inner defiance*. This is like driving with the brakes on. You're slowly moving forward but stopping yourself at the same time. It makes everything more difficult than it needs to be and leads to third chakra exhaustion.

It's not that the will is completely broken. Endurers can be very stubborn. It's as if their arms are crossed over their chest, their feet grounded into the earth, and their body is saying: "You can't make me," yet outwardly they are resigned to doing it anyway.

Autonomy becomes the driving quest for people with this pattern. Having been robbed of it, they unconsciously seek it in most situations, especially relationships. Because they can't say a direct *no* very easily, they tend to say *yes*, and then whine about it later. "Do you want to go to the movies?" If they say *no*, the other person pushes and says, "Oh, come on, it will be fun!" Then they give in and say *yes*, but later complain that they didn't like the movie. They feel pushed, then resist. And, of course, when one resists, the people around them push even more, which creates more resistance in a vicious cycle.

If you can't let your charge out (because it is shamed or punished), then you have to learn to keep all that charge inside. In order to store the charge you can't release, the body has to create more insulation between the inner world and the outer, and more tissue to store the charge. This can show up as weight problems, muscle and joint stiffness, and a body that is hard to enliven.

With a pattern of holding in, they may contain a lot of blocked charge, yet outwardly they seem calm and steady. It's just not their nature to be big, flamboyant, or expressive. Their process is deeply internal, and they hate exposure or invasion of their privacy.

With so much energy packed into the third chakra and stuck there, other parts of the body are robbed of energy. Their butt may be tucked under and tight, constricting the first two chakras, the shoulders rounded and the head forward. It's as if the upper chakras and the lower ones meet and conflict in the belly area, where the charge gets fixated.

Because the charge builds up inside, there is a longing to let it out—a longing that is simultaneously feared and resisted.

Sometimes, after enduring a situation for too long, they erupt in anger or tears, no longer able to put up with it. This is actually a breakthrough, though the one receiving this outburst might not see it so favorably.

It's not like this structure is undercharged like the Oral pattern or has a charge that's split like the Schizoid pattern. They are not absent of feelings or even of charge, though it's typically not visible on the outside. Instead they are masters at self-concealment, safely hiding their true feelings, even from themselves. Alone, they may brood, seeing themselves as a victim, but outwardly you might think they were rather numb. The suffering is buried on the inside, with one who feels alone and trapped inside the defense he developed to keep himself safe.

Recognize the Pattern When:

- You become sullen and resentful.
- Being in a charged situation makes you shut down and be still.
- You make your body dense.
- You feel yourself digging in your heels with: "You can't make me."
- You resist everything, even your own urges.
- You sabotage your goals.
- Your critic becomes a monologue inside your head.
- You blame others for your reality.

Gifts of the Endurer Pattern

The gifts of the Endurer structure are many. As you remember, personality traits develop in childhood by finding what "works" in a given situation. That trait later turns out to be an asset, even though it may have its cost. The good news is this: as we work through the issues of each character pattern, we reduce the cost, but we don't lose the gifts.

Loyalty. With this character pattern, you'll find someone who is grounded and solid, probably the most grounded of any of the structures. If you were to hire someone for a job, especially a job that needs to be done meticulously, you would want to hire an Endurer, as they are loyal and steady. They will stick with the task, show up regularly, and do the work. As clients, I found that Endurers would faithfully come to therapy on time each week; they would participate to the extent of their capacity and make slow but steady progress.

Diplomacy. Endurers don't make a lot of trouble or drama and generally get along well with others. They prefer to be left alone and assume others are the same, so they don't demand much of other people. They tolerate others' quirks more than the average person and are often peacemakers who can be highly diplomatic, even with difficult people. *They are experts at putting up with difficulty but terrible at changing it.*

Inner strength. Sometimes called the strong, silent type, they are not easily budged or pushed. This may seem contradictory, as we are talking about someone whose will was thwarted. But even though they don't move forward easily with their own will, they do resist being pushed around by others—precisely because that was their experience in the past. Therefore, they maintain their ground, with a kind of resolute strength that can at times seem stubborn. Think of them as stoic.

Pleasing. Endurers care what others think of them, and they want to be liked. Caught in a conflict between being themselves and pleasing others, they sincerely want to please others. So they will endeavor to do the best they can, even as their inner critic constantly points out where they come up short. They are generally good to their friends and loved ones—but they don't overdo it like the Oral structure.

Healing the Endurer Pattern

I remember a young woman I worked with for about six months who carried this structure. Even though she showed up faithfully week after week, it didn't seem like we were making much progress. Two years later, she wrote me a letter saying how much those six months had changed her life. I shook my head in wonder, thinking, "Well, you could have fooled me!"

The tricky thing about healing the Endurer pattern is that their need for autonomy makes them inwardly resist the helper, even as they appear to comply outwardly. You give them an exercise to do during the week and they don't do it. Or they do the exercise without really engaging in it, then tell you it doesn't work. They often feel a kind of triumph in getting others to fail.

Healing the Endurer character structure takes time and patience. They rarely do things quickly. They don't go for big catharsis, but rather take slow and steady incremental steps forward. They have a hard time getting started, but once they move in a direction, they keep on with it.

Here are some tactics that are helpful for the healing process:

Playfulness. I use laughter, teasing, and play with this pattern. It helps overcome their heavy seriousness, takes them off guard, and begins to loosen things up. Many of the bioenergetic exercises in this book can be used as a form of play—minimizing the need to perform and maximizing a positive experience.

Don't be invested in a particular outcome. When working with this pattern, I suggest things in a tangential, even paradoxical manner: "Well, some people find this exercise helpful, but that's probably not your style." That gives them the freedom to differentiate and say, "Yes, I do want to try that," because it's phrased in a way that it doesn't feel like they have to. Therapists call this *paradoxical intervention*, assigning the opposite of what you want to happen, so that the client resists and participates in what might be good for them.

Expand choices. Endurers tend to see themselves as having no choice about their circumstances. It's not helpful to list those choices, saying, "Well, you could have done this," or, "Why didn't you do that?" That only brings up resistance, and they are probably telling themselves that already. Instead, invite them to list other interpretations of a situation, other possible avenues of behavior, and generally expand their range of what's possible, even listing things that are unrealistic. This combats the sense of hopelessness and develops an important skill.

Tease complaints into anger and action. Because Endurers feel trapped and stuck, they tend to complain. I consider whining to be like that smoldering fire, but one that can flare up when a little air is blown on it. A comment made lightly, like, "Oh, come on, it isn't really that bad is it?" can provoke an enraged response, which for Endurers is actually a good thing. This brings the charge level up and gives you something to work with. If they can feel their charge, they can begin to feel their power.

Once the anger surfaces it can be directed toward action. That action can be hitting the couch with a bat and expressing anger, writing in a journal all the things you haven't been able to say, or strategizing how to take steps to change a situation.

Encourage acts of autonomy. There's an exercise I sometimes do in my workshops, where all the participants line up in two rows, facing each other. I give the command to one side to say, "No," and the other side to say, "Yes," with both sides using their body as well as their voice. It very quickly escalates into a shouting match, then reaches a certain pitch where everyone starts laughing and hugging each other. Then, of course, I have the two lines switch roles, where the Nos can say, "Yes," and the Yeses can say, "No."

Tug-of-War Exercise

You've heard about the inner child? Well, this exercise invites you to regress into your inner "brat." This awakens the unbridled feeling of childish power that got thwarted at a young age and energizes the third chakra.

(This exercise requires two people and cannot be done alone.)

Grab a yoga strap or a large towel or blanket that you can twist into a long rope. Each person grabs an end to the "rope," then stands facing their partner, as far away as the length of the rope.

Each person is invited to think about something that is important to them—something they don't want to have taken away. It can be their fire, their sexuality, or their freedom, or they can even imagine something as simple as a toy.

On a count of three, each person begins pulling the rope, reverting to the feelings and actions of a three-year-old. They yell out, "Give it to me! This is mine! I want it!" or whatever comes to mind. Allow this feeling to come into the body as you ground into your feet to avoid getting pushed over.

Allow the energy of your inner brat to come out. When he or she has had her say, you can stop and take time to feel your third chakra and your charge in general.

Will Exercise

This exercise also involves two people, though one facilitates for the other. We'll call the facilitator Person A and the participant Person B.

Person B thinks about something he or she needs to do with their will. Examples would be sticking to a diet, finishing a project, maintaining a yoga practice, or getting to bed earlier. It should be something the person finds challenging.

When this is clear, Person B starts with grounding and takes a solid stance, pushing down into the earth. She then brings her arms alongside her body, with elbows straight and hands in a fist, backs of the wrists facing outward.

The facilitator, Person A, applies a small amount of pressure to the backs of the wrists while Person B tries to lift her arms, *keeping her elbows straight.*

The amount of pressure is enough to make Person B have to work hard to raise her arms, but not so much pressure that she can't do so. When the arms tremble, you know that they are running some charge.

When the wrists lift up to shoulder height, Person A lets go. The result is a feeling of breakthrough, with the charge moving upward through the third chakra.

chapter 22

the
CHALLENGER-
DEFENDER
STRUCTURE

||||||||||||||||||||||||||||||||||||||||||||||||||||||||||||||||||||||||||||||||

The Power Broker

Cameron was the kind of guy who stood out in any crowd. Tall and handsome, broad-shouldered and boisterous, he had a commanding, charismatic presence. His confidence, intelligence, and warmth gave him the aura of someone who would be your champion and always protect you, yet his high charge and powerful demeanor were a bit intimidating. It was easy to be both charmed and disarmed by him at the same time.

He worked as an attorney, specializing in corporate and environmental law, wanting to serve a cause that benefited the planet. His passion was to be a voice for indigenous people who were exploited by corporate interests. His firm was large, his work complex and demanding, sending him to remote parts of the world as an advocate for the underdog.

Even in his personal life, he was drawn to protecting the meek, reflected in his marriage to Jeanette, a beautiful woman 18 years his junior. She was a devoted partner but had little sense of her own power. (You might say she was a combination of the

Oral and Endurer character structures, which often go well with this pattern.)

His wife, however, revealed to me another side of Cameron that wasn't so benevolent. When she tried to talk about anything amiss in their relationship, the same man that she saw as a protector suddenly became her challenger. He would get angry and defensive over the slightest hint of criticism, with little tolerance for her hurt emotions. He had even less patience for the weakness of those closest to him, his kids included, with an attitude of: "Just pull yourself together." While he wasn't physically abusive, the charge of his anger was feared by his wife and children, who tiptoed around him.

His wife also told me that even though he was the head of a successful law firm, he had few, if any, close friends. His need for power was so absolute that anyone who challenged him was summarily dismissed. Since his co-workers couldn't confront him about anything, they instead talked behind his back, vilifying him for his dominating and aggressive behavior. To Cameron, it seemed like everyone was against him. Feeling alone against the world, he could justify his calloused treatment of others.

It may seem contradictory that he would champion the underdog yet insist on absolute power in his work and relationships, but this is the paradox of the Challenger-Defender structure. They will defend the meek but challenge anyone who dares to thwart their power. They can move from savior to enemy so fast it makes your head spin.

The Challenger-Defender Source of Wounding

While the classic name for this type is *Psychopath* (which describes a more extreme form), other names invoke more compassion, such as the Used Child, the Betrayed Child, or the Aggressive pattern. Typically, there was a past betrayal that was so hurtful that he lost trust in anything larger than himself. It seemed that no one cared, and certainly no one could be trusted. In Cameron's case, his father had died of a gang-related murder, and his mother worked two jobs, leaving him alone to care for his younger brother and sister.

The Betrayed or Used Child can sometimes result from sexual abuse, where the family doesn't know, or even worse, doesn't care about the torment the child experiences. It happens to children who are used for their parents' needs—to cover up alcoholism, to deny physical abuse, or to work for the family at too young an age. One client I had was used as a decoy as his family escaped Nazi Germany along the front lines. He was only five years old at the time. Another had to sell newspapers on the street at age ten because his father drank all the money away. A young woman I worked with had spent her childhood caring for a mentally ill single mother, who constantly berated her, yet as an only child, she had nowhere to turn. It can even be a wounding that happens later in life, such as a woman I knew who had been raped at gunpoint when she was 16.

Unlike the Endurer, whose wounding arrests development at the early stage of the third chakra (18 months to 3 years), the Challenger-Defender does complete this stage, developing their power and will, only to get thwarted in the heart chakra.

The feeling of betrayal comes from adults overpowering the child's newly found sense of power. Often the betrayal is so severe that the child, whether consciously or unconsciously, decides he *will do whatever it takes* to make sure he is never vulnerable again. In more pathological cases, this whatever-it-takes attitude can be deceitful, manipulative, and downright criminal, with little sense of conscience, which is why this pattern has been classically called the Psychopath. I prefer to avoid this term, since many people who exhibit this pattern are far from the scoundrels who embezzle funds or molest little children. They are simply people who gravitate toward positions of power and avoid vulnerability. Some, like Cameron, use their power to do good, yet still intimidate or dominate others.

Unlike the Masochist, who runs an intense inner critic, the Challenger-Defender criticizes everyone else but cannot tolerate being criticized in return. It's very common that they have one set of rules for themselves and another for others. A man may be very jealous and possessive, even while he is having a secret affair.

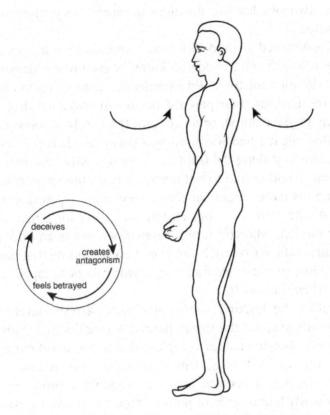

Figure 13 Challenger-Defender Character Structure:
Strong, defensive, energy held up in shoulders and head

Charge Pattern

People with this pattern are able to handle high charge and direct it with precision. They are comfortable with power, even thrive on it. They excel at jobs in which they command others: CEOs, army generals, politicians, police, and even clergy. Many become lawyers or therapists. If you want a therapist who will support you through your most vulnerable moments, this type will give you undivided attention. But criticize them for an item on the bill or any other conduct, and your champion can turn on you in the blink of an eye, accusing you of having the problem instead.

One of the defenses of this pattern is to inflate their body with their charge in order to seem bigger than they are. The torso appears puffed up like a blowfish, either wide shoulders and puffed-out chest, or women with large breasts and puffy shoulders, out of proportion with their lower body. But this character also inflates his résumé and tells tall tales to make the story better. They have commanding eyes and a head that often tips slightly forward, almost as if they are looking down on everyone.

Their charge is carried mostly in the upper torso, while the lower body remains loose and flowing. They can be sexually seductive charmers, even predatory, yet sex is more about power and excitement than an experience of intimacy. Often, they suffer from tight shoulders and neck, as they command their charge largely through the throat chakra, becoming strong orators who can manipulate others through persuasive conversation. In this aspect, they make good salespeople as well.

Challenger-Defenders often take their prodigious amount of charge and direct it toward other people. Undercharged people respond to this, as they receive someone's potent, undivided attention. On the negative side, however, Challengers can direct explosive anger toward their children, partner, or co-workers, with little comprehension of how it feels to be on the receiving end. After the outburst, the Challenger's charge is more regulated, and they suddenly become more loving and easygoing. They quickly forget what happened and assume the other person has also let it go—even though this is rarely the case.

Recognize the Pattern When:

- You feel like everyone's against you.
- You can't ask for help.
- You're too quick to fight.
- You are dominating or intimidating others.
- You feel like you have to do it all alone.

- No one's on your side.

- You can't be vulnerable.

Gifts of the Challenger-Defender Pattern

While it's easy to demonize people with this pattern, their gifts are many. For this reason, others often put up with their shadow side, because the rewards of status, success, and money often go with the package. The wife gets the big house, the prestigious partner, and the strong protector. The husband gets to lie back while his powerhouse wife handles the children, a demanding job, and their social life—as long as he is willing to have it her way.

Highly capable. If you want someone to argue your case as a defense attorney, the Challenger-Defender will be determined to win at all costs. Their strong charge makes them very capable, able to handle big challenges and get things done. They hold up well in a crisis and easily turn their energy into action. They handle their difficult tasks without complaint. (In fact, they despise whiners who play the victim.) They rarely do anything they don't want to do and put full force into what they choose to do.

Loving and protective. People with this pattern can also be extremely loving when they feel their gifts are valued or needed, especially when they have the safety of holding an upper edge, such as being older or more experienced. These are the strong protectors women swoon over, the knight in shining armor who comes to their rescue, or the overprotective mother.

Innovative. Since they are not bound by other people's rules, they are great innovators. Steve Jobs, who ran Apple and created the iPhone, is a classic example. He was known to be dictatorial and often coldhearted, yet he innovated a technology that changed the world.

Strong leadership. When healthy, Challengers make strong leaders, good at motivating and commanding others. They can run companies, armies, and even countries. They have strong verbal skills and can outargue almost anyone. They are often tireless crusaders who won't quit until their cause is won. Most politicians have a fair amount of this structure. Both Bernie Sanders and Donald Trump exhibited this pattern and were able to motivate large crowds with their charge, though with vastly different agendas.

Optimistic. While cheerfulness wouldn't quite describe the Challenger, they are generally optimistic with a can-do attitude that can be impulsive. Refusing to see themselves as victims, they rarely get depressed over a situation. Instead, they take action to change it and refuse to quit until they have solved the problem. In this way, they are quite the opposite of the Endurer, who puts up with things rather than make change.

Healing the Challenger-Defender Pattern

Challenger-Defenders aren't the kind of people who typically show up for therapy or workshops. That requires vulnerability, which they generally avoid. Often, they don't even see that they have a problem, and they certainly wouldn't trust someone else to solve it for them.

Usually it's a partner who brings them in for healing, or it might be the loss of a relationship. They love deeply and can be fiercely loyal, so when loss occurs—as it often does for someone who dominates—they may even put their healing in the category of "whatever it takes" to regain their sense of power and equilibrium. They don't take rejection lightly.

What's important to remember is that this powerful person was a betrayed child, and the betrayal was severe. It's essential to let them know you are on their side, that you see their point of view, and that you appreciate what it took for them to get through their difficulties. They need someone to be a champion for them so they can let go of having to fight for themselves.

Compassion, rather than confrontation, is the best approach. As they gain compassion for themselves, they gradually learn to have compassion for others. As they learn how they were overpowered, they can begin to understand how their anger and forcefulness overpower others. They must learn to temper their outbursts and understand that others are different than they are. Not all people want to be powerful or live in the limelight.

As the defense pattern begins to break down, there is often an incredible vulnerability underneath. It must be understood that this is a very delicate stage, in which the healing process can proceed forward or become derailed. Challengers will test their therapist endlessly, to make sure he or she can be trusted. One must be patient with this and remain steady, strong, and trustworthy.

In relationships, they actually trust someone who can stand up to them more than someone they can dominate. If a partner stands up for their rights, they win points and respect. If they criticize and whine, it merely provokes more of the defense. So when dealing with this type, stand powerfully in your ground, channel your charge carefully, and ask for what you want, rather than complain about what you're not getting. This is good advice, in any case, but especially when dealing with the intimidating power of the Challenger-Defender.

Reflection Exercise

1. Imagine a time when you felt alone and perhaps betrayed by circumstances or someone you loved. What were the feelings at the time? Hold yourself in compassion.

2. If someone had been there for you as a champion, someone real or imagined, who would it have been? What would they have done to protect you?

3. Imagine this more positive scenario happening to the child you were at the time, with this champion at your back. Notice what it feels like to have that kind of support. Notice how it can allow you to soften and return to some of the innocence of a child.

chapter 23

the RIGID CHARACTER STRUCTURE

||||||||||||||||||||||||||||||||||||||||||||||||||||||||||||||||||||||||||||||||

The Achiever

Where would we be without people who exhibit the Rigid character structure? For they are the ones who keep everything in order, make things sparkle with cleanliness, get the work done, and somehow always manage to look good while they're at it. Model citizens of the culture, they are bright, attractive, friendly, and obedient to the rules. Often the envy of others, they are the graduate with honors from the best schools, the high-paid executive with the fancy car, the performer with a cadre of fans, or the beauty queen who makes men swoon. Little do people understand that they too have a hidden suffering.

Veronica was a perfect example of the Rigid pattern, and "perfect" might be the best way to describe her. Physically, she was a beauty, with a slightly muscular build, bright sparkling eyes, and a full head of dark, wavy hair that never seemed to be out of place. She dressed impeccably and always gave the impression of being well put together. When she sat down in the office, she placed her purse carefully on the side table, each time in the same place, took off her shoes and set them neatly beside each other, and sat up straight like a pet that's waiting to be patted on the head with the words "Good girl."

As she began to tell me about herself, she listed her many accomplishments: a Harvard degree in business and a well-paying job as an assistant to a high-ranking executive. She had three children between the ages of 6 and 11, and she gave them every opportunity to engage in sports and extracurricular activities. Yet she feared she wasn't a "good enough" mother because her nanny drove them around when she was working. She had what she called a "good" marriage but couldn't give much detail of what was good about it. Her husband was a physician, and they lived in a beautiful house in an elegant suburb of a major city, but both were so hardworking they didn't spend much time together.

When I asked her why she was here, she told me that she had put on 20 pounds since her last child and wanted to know what she could do about it. She thought maybe body-oriented therapy might help. It seemed she wanted to enlist my services to become even more perfect.

As often happens with someone like this, I first wonder what she is doing in my office—this person seems so much more together than I—as if she already has it all figured out. But that is the issue: *she has to be perfect,* and herein lies the pain of this structure.

The Rigid Structure Source of Wounding

All children need to be loved and appreciated. Under normal conditions, this allows a child to develop a healthy sense of self, to be able to relate to others and form solid, loving relationships later in life. But for the child who develops the Rigid pattern, the love he or she received was conditional. They were loved if they did things right, and rejected if they made a mistake, broke the rules, or failed to perform. Too much emphasis was placed on outer performance and too little on inner experience. One's identity gets fused with performance rather than the interior self.

This is the child who is sent to her room when she acts up and told to come out *only* when she can act the way she's supposed to. This is the child who is highly praised for being precocious, while her mistakes and insecurities are not tolerated. This is the child who grows up with very definite rules and expectations and is rewarded when those expectations are met, but gets rejected when the childish and messy aspects of her personality show up.

As a result, the child doesn't get to finish the more immature stages of early childhood and instead has to "hurry up" to become a little adult. Their inner emotional life is not seen, reflected, or responded to, so it gets pushed down into the shadow world—hidden from consciousness, with the fear that it might erupt at any moment and bring shame. The blocked emotional charge is then channeled into achievement and performance, at which they excel. And just as it was with their parents, the culture also rewards them for their achievements, further widening the gap between the inner, authentic self and their outer performance.

The Rigid character structure results from a childhood that goes reasonably well during its early stages. The child gets a good sense of his own body and grounding in chakra one and learns that he belongs in the world. He is nurtured and played with, as appropriate, in his second chakra stage, along with support for his emotions. He develops his will and autonomy in the third chakra stage, without being betrayed or overpowered. He even makes it to the heart chakra stage, where he starts to shape his personality to win love and approval. But here is where the wounding happens.

Classically, the age of wounding occurs between three and a half and five years of age, though later situations can also contribute to this pattern. This is the time when a child has enough physical and neurological maturity to have mastered impulse control and have good language skills. But after being emotionally nurtured in their younger stages, they suddenly have to put away their childish impulses and "behave" like an older, more mature child, hence the alternate name of the "Hurried Child."

Maybe they have younger brothers and sisters who have now been born, and they can no longer act like the baby of the family. Maybe a boy child starts school and discovers he can't cry without being labeled a sissy. I was the baby in my family, with a big age gap between me and my two older brothers. My parents didn't push me, but I *pushed myself* to grow up, so as to be accepted by my brothers (which didn't work!).

Often the parents pass on their own Rigid structure, thinking they are helping their child by teaching him to follow the rules and correcting his behavior. They show their love by pushing their child to be the best they can possibly be, thinking they are doing them a favor. And in some ways they are, for achievement is definitely rewarded in today's world, with money, prestige, and admiration.

One of my clients was a prominent physician and best-selling author. He claimed he owed his success to the time his father beat him so mercilessly for a bad grade in high school that he never dared to fail again. From that point on, he worked extra hard and was admitted into a good medical school and carried his discipline through the many years of his training. He later tried to enforce his son to take the same route, albeit unsuccessfully. Finally he came to realize how abusive his father had been and then could see how he was passing a version of that down to his son.

Steven Kessler, author of *The 5 Personality Patterns*, points out that a Rigid character structure can also arise from a family in which there was a lot of chaos and confusion. Often, out of sheer survival, a child may take it upon herself to be the one who creates and maintains some type of order or normalcy, just for the sake of her own sanity. This then becomes both a useful skill and a gilded prison.

With emphasis on outer performance, the child loses touch with his or her true, authentic self. There is no room to make a mistake or to be less than perfect. Like Veronica, one can't have a bad hair day or gain a little weight. This is the tragedy that no one sees, including the Rigid herself. Instead, it's taken as normal to live under the gun of constantly high expectations.

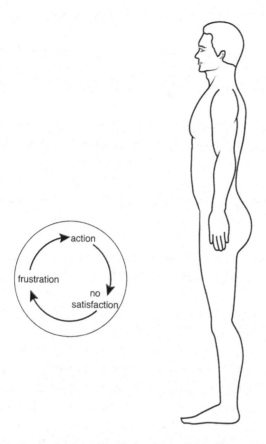

**Figure 14 Rigid Character Structure: Well proportioned,
tight in chest, held back in middle. Arches and leans forward.**

Charge Pattern

Those who exhibit the Rigid pattern have the highest charge
of any of the character structures mentioned thus far. They dis-
tribute that charge evenly throughout their body and limbs, but
more toward the surface of the body—the muscles and the skin—
while the deep self remains a mystery. Their eyes are sparkly,
their conversation animated, and they seldom hold still for long,

needing to keep moving to handle the tremendous charge that is always present.

They are happiest in action. In fact, the Rigid can be extremely restless when there's nothing to do. But that happens rarely. Since nothing is ever quite good enough, it can always be perfected a little more.

Their bodies are neither fat nor thin, but tend to be medium build, muscular and fit, with a high metabolism. They go for athletics in high school and college and generally keep up some kind of physical activity as an adult, whether it's playing racquetball, dancing, or just running or working out. One person I knew ran several miles, six days a week, for years. He wore out his hips before he stopped.

As the name Rigid might suggest, their bodies are less flexible than others, even though they are highly athletic. Many go to yoga to improve their flexibility but adhere to rigid repetitious routines that further bind the charge, rather than using yoga to relax more deeply and listen to their body.

Emotions—at least the messy ones that won't fit onto a Hallmark greeting card—are repressed in this structure. Instead that charge is channeled into activity: compulsively working, cleaning, organizing, exercising, or getting things done in general. Their pattern with others is to hold back emotionally. If you're in a relationship with a Rigid, you can never quite tell what he or she is feeling. They are rarely the first one to say, "I love you," nor are they likely to share their needs, deepest desires, or insecurities.

Because the emotional realm is repressed, they don't check into their inner feelings to see what they really want—in fact, they doubt their right to want at all. Instead they figure out what they are "supposed to do" and shape themselves accordingly. If they look at a menu, they don't scan for what they're hungry for, but what fits their calorie protocol for the day. If they shop for clothing, they pick what looks good over what feels more comfortable. If they wonder whether to do something, it's not the pleasure that is attractive but whether it serves their purpose of achievement in some way. You might say they are a bit narcissistic, but it is only their deep doubt that they can be loved for their imperfect selves that fuels the narcissism. They are actually quite capable of caring deeply for others.

Whereas the Schizoid structure has a split between mind and body, the Rigid structure has a split between the inner, authentic self and the outer, performing self. Their charge then is understandably channeled into the performing self, which becomes further charged from the rewards that come from the outside world, thus perpetuating the split. The glory is that they can succeed. The tragedy is that they have to.

Inevitably, something happens in their life that destroys their thin veneer of perfection. They lose their fortune in the stock market, they get caught in a sexual scandal, their marriage fails, or they get some kind of injury that prevents them from performing. They gain weight, get wrinkles, or experience a loss somewhere.

And when this happens, they crash, feeling devastated and lost, because so much of their identity is caught up in their image. When they come to therapy, it is often to learn how to fix it again—how to lose that 40 pounds they put on, how to get their fortune back, how to fix their marriage. Such failures are a golden opportunity to make contact with the real and vulnerable self underneath. Do not enable them in their addiction to perfection, but gently look for what is aching to emerge and be seen.

Recognize the Pattern When:

- You are trying to be perfect.

- You're always looking for what's wrong in yourself or others.

- You're trying to help others (partner, child, friends) be more perfect when they haven't asked for it.

- You're upset when there's disorder or things are out of place.

- You can't act until you know what the rules are.

- You're ignoring your feelings to follow the rules.

- You doubt your right to want and need.

Gifts of the Rigid Pattern

The gifts in this pattern are many, as they are the envy of most everyone around them. In fact, most people would call them gifted! Rigid types look good, play well with others, and keep things running smoothly. They are attractive, fit, and pleasant to look at and be around. They are highly disciplined, keep their agreements, and can always be counted on to do their best. Rigids are generally bright and cheerful (almost to the exclusion of other emotions).

Clean and organized. You can count on a Rigid type to keep things clean and sparkling. They love order and structure. Clothes are neatly folded in their drawers. Their desktops are attractive and functional. It seems there's always a Rigid in my workshops who needs the exercises spelled out step by step, who wants to know the exact time the break will occur and frequently calls me over to make sure she is "doing it right." As a more fluid Oral character myself, I actually appreciate the invitation to create more structure.

Energetic and cheerful. Rigid-patterned people rarely seem to run out of energy. If they get depressed, they rarely show it and might not even know it themselves. They have a positive outlook on life that moves forward easily. They don't dwell on negativity from the past.

Reliable. You can count on Rigid types to do things right and to do things well. They are the model citizen, the hard worker, and the one who perseveres in difficult tasks, always pursuing excellence.

Accomplished. Rigids love to accomplish things. They have a long list to brag about, many of which make wonderful contributions to society. They inspire others to reach higher and accomplish as well. They have what it takes to get through medical school, rise to the top of their company, or compete in demanding sports. They are certainly the boyfriend or girlfriend you want to bring home to your parents.

Healing the Rigid Pattern

Rigids tend to seek help when something happens to crack the outer perfection, but their interest can be more oriented to self-improvement than self-inquiry. With a slight shift in framework, you can help the "fallen Rigid" discover that the failure to live up to their own and others' expectations is actually the gateway to their healing. Direct the inquiry toward discovery of the authentic being that dwells within.

Letting go of what they *should do,* they can better ask what they *want to do.* This is best accomplished through making contact with the inner flow of feelings and emotion. At first, this may be a complete mystery. After all, they haven't had the luxury of inquiring into their own needs for a very long time, if ever. It takes a while to begin sorting out the many repressed emotions that were pushed into the shadows of the psyche and feel their own unique desire.

Because this structure was the Hurried Child, it's important to let them take their time. They don't drop down into their emotions quickly or easily. In my workshops, when a person with this structure volunteers to work in front of the class, they almost always worry that they're taking up too much of the group's time. On the contrary, the whole group is learning from their experience.

By helping a Rigid see that the rules they try so hard to obey are just an arbitrary set of standards, they can ask the inner soul for direction instead. Often what first emerges are the shadowy emotions. By definition, our shadow represents the aspects of our personality that we reject or suppress. When the shadow is pointed out by a friend or partner, as it inevitably is, one's first reaction is to defend against it, using denial, distraction, or any other way to keep it at bay. It's important to accept and reflect these emotions in a positive way and allow them to be reclaimed as an aspect of the authentic self.

A clue to identifying the shadow qualities lies in looking at what we judge in others, those traits that really get our charge going, such as someone who is a slob, irresponsible, overly sexual, or self-centered. Usually that trait is something the judging person wasn't allowed to do, so the judgment is a kind of jealousy. While the point is not to become a raging bitch just because we weren't allowed to be angry, there is a movement toward wholeness when we can reclaim our shadow consciously, rather than have it run us unconsciously.

In some of my workshops, I have people *dance* their shadow, bringing the rejected energies to the surface through movement. Each person takes some moments in the center, acting out the bitch, the tyrant, the slut, the slob, the prima donna, or the needy child. After each person takes their turn, the whole group is laughing and more bonded with one another than before. Students quickly learn that they are less likely to be judged when their shadow comes out than when they keep it hidden. Once we know a person's shadow, we can better trust them.

You know a Rigid is healing when they can access their emotions, when they know what they truly want, when they can open to intimacy and allow themselves to make mistakes. The hardest thing is for them to accept themselves as ordinary, just like everyone else, and to realize that achievement is not the measure of the soul. When they can laugh at themselves, they are well on their way.

Reflection Exercise

On the left side of a piece of paper list all the characteristics you developed as a child in order to be "good." Maybe you were quiet, neat, helpful, responsible, or the straight-A student. Just write a word or two for each quality.

Next to each item on the list, down the right-hand side, name what you had to give up in order to develop those traits. If you wrote down *reserved*, you might have had to give up being needy or emotional. If you wrote down *quiet*, you might have had to give up being noisy. If you were neat, you had to give up being messy.

Next, imagine yourself doing or being some of the things on the right-hand list. Notice whether it brings up charge for you. Track your charge to see where it is in the body and any feelings or emotions.

Authentic Movement

It is good for the Rigid character to find their authentic self, in body, mind, and spirit. This exercise helps to free the body. Set aside about 20 minutes.

Take some time where you can be with yourself, wearing comfortable clothes, with some empty floor space in which to move around freely. Close your eyes and feel into your body. Notice any movements your body might want to make, and allow them to happen, slowly at first, starting with subtle micromovements around the core. As you continue to focus on the smaller movements, very gradually allow them to get bigger. Eventually allow them to get as big as they want, even adding any sound that wants to come out. Allow the movements to express your charge from deep within. The movements may change from one thing to another or from one body part to another. You might curl up in a ball or stamp your feet into the ground. Just see what emerges.

When the larger movements have been fully expressed, gradually begin to tone it down into subtler movements again, until you come to a natural stopping place.

Allow at least 10 minutes or longer for the movements. If it is shorter, you are hurrying too much. Go back and try it again. Use music if you like, but make sure the music doesn't have a rhythm that dictates your movement.

When you are finished moving, take the rest of the time to write in your journal, draw a picture, or engage in some form of expression.

Make sure the movement comes from within the body, not what you are "supposed" to do. Avoid dance moves, yoga postures, martial arts *katas*, or anything that has a fixed form. See what emerges organically from your own body.

part v

RELATIONSHIP
and
SOCIETY

chapter 24

CHARGE

and

RELATIONSHIPS

||||||||||||||||||||||||||||||||||||||||||||||||||||||||||||||||||||||||||||||||||||||||||||||||||||||||

How to Keep It Cool
and Hot at the Same Time

*There is always some madness in love. But there
is also always some reason in madness.*

FRIEDRICH NIETZSCHE

It was a tender moment between Charles and Janet. They gazed at each other with moist eyes, and their hearts were soft. They tenderly hugged and held each other, opening to a new and fresh intimacy.

But a few moments earlier, their charge was sky-high. Angry shouts and accusations were flying between them like a high-powered tennis match. Janet was able to hold her ground, but she did so by locking down on her charge, arms folded over her chest in stubborn resistance. With a strong tendency toward the Endurer pattern, she was good at sitting on her charge—to a point. But when something pushed beyond her limit, she would erupt.

Charles, on the other hand, was a highly charged person prone to the Rigid pattern, with a slight dose of Challenger-Defender that would emerge in tense situations. He was strongly invested in the idea that there was a right and wrong way to do things and quick to point out when he thought Janet was wrong. At the same time, he was highly sensitive to anything that remotely resembled criticism. Even with Janet's careful phrasing of words, he could react defensively, his charge shooting up so quickly that he was unable to hear what she was saying.

When they weren't getting triggered, Charles and Janet had a strong charge of attraction between them. They were dedicated partners, very much in love, but they kept getting trapped in a counterproductive charge pattern they were unable to break.

In the session, I encouraged each of them to focus on the charge in their own body rather than on what the other was doing, or even the story they were telling themselves. One at a time, I helped them listen more closely to their feelings and look for what deeper issues might be getting triggered from their own past. Then I used mild physical exercises to help some emotional expression without the other immediately responding. After each of them had discharged sufficiently, they could finally listen to each other with empathy, and a sense of intimacy was restored. Now the charge was bringing them closer, rather than pushing them apart.

All relationships deal with charge in some way. Whether it's the charge of attraction and sexuality that pulls us together or the charge of getting triggered that pulls us apart, relationships are a crucible for learning to handle charge.

The way charge flows through an individual is the building block. That's where we start. But we are not isolated beings. We interact with other people who also have charge. We interact with groups, we interact with children, co-workers, authority figures, and intimate partners. Our own patterns are constantly triggered by the charge of others.

Sometimes those patterns fit like an exquisitely choreographed dance. One person takes a step and the other reacts with a counterstep. This can be good or bad, healthy or unhealthy. We may feel that wonderful "Ah" when we're with the other person, feeling completed by them. The juicy charge of attraction keeps us *in* relationship, but it can also have a dark side. We can be brought down by this dance, when our own dysfunctional patterns raise their ugly heads in reaction to another—sometimes over and over again. One person's aggression makes the other shrink back with fear. One person's needs overwhelm their partner, who becomes even more withholding. Someone who is addicted to a substance is often "perfectly" paired with a co-dependent enabler. Sometimes we feel a strong spark with someone, while with others there is no spark at all. Still others might make us feel irritated every time we're around them.

So when we bring the concept of charge into relationships, it gets very complex and could easily be a book of its own. Yet it is essential to understand charge in order to navigate the changing tides of relationship. After mastering our own charge, our next challenge is to allow that charge to dance with another.

Energy Fields Overlap

Everything has an energy field. While charge flows through our own body, it also emanates into the field around us. Invisible to most, this field overlaps with the fields of others when we are in close proximity. In ways we don't yet understand, this influence can even occur at a distance, as evidenced by the numerous studies on healing and distant prayer.[1]

This means we can be unconsciously influenced by the energy fields of others, both one-on-one and in crowds or work situations. We often say we like someone's "vibes" or that we feel heavy or uplifted around different people. Students or devotees of a guru have been known to receive profound awakenings, just by being in the presence of the master, even when no words or physical touch are exchanged. Just because we can't "see" these fields doesn't mean they don't affect us. We can become aware of them by noticing what happens to our own charge.

Charge Wants to Find Balance

Not only does charge try to balance within us, through a natural flow of charging and discharging, it also tries to balance between two people or within a group or family. I remember years ago when I had four kids at home, my husband would come home from work at the end of the day, often grumpy from the stress of his job. But he wasn't prone to expressing his anger, except through a moodiness that pervaded the house. Inevitably, on those days, one of the kids would try to provoke him. They would repeatedly do something annoying until he finally discharged with a quick burst of, "That's enough! Now stop it!" Once that happened, the energy in the field was discharged, and everyone would settle down. The charge had balanced out. It was as if the kids sensed his pent-up charge and unconsciously acted out to release it.

In general, I notice that higher-charge people and lower-charge people tend to be attracted to one another. The one with lower charge feels energized and uplifted by the one who carries a higher charge. It makes them feel alive and inspires them to action. The depressed person may feel listless when alone but brighten up around someone who is energized. Even someone's anger can wake us up when we're feeling lethargic, though not always in the best way.

By contrast, the higher-charge person feels more relaxed around someone who carries less charge. There is more freedom and ease. A high-charge executive, for example, wants to settle down at the end of the day. Comfort might be more important to him than stimulation. When he comes home to a pack of noisy kids jumping up and down, he doesn't get to relax, and his charge is more likely to be released on the kids, just as it was for my husband.

Just as various chemicals bond together because of the electrostatic attraction between their atoms, people have bonding patterns as well. In the short run, these bonding patterns seem to bring a positive result, but in the long run, they may become annoying or even damaging. Over time, the low-charge person can feel exhausted trying to keep up with their high-charge partner—simply because they don't have enough of their own energy. They might find themselves thinking, "Why can't you ever relax? You have to go, go, go, all the time, and I'm so tired of it! I just want to stay home for a night and watch TV."

The high-charge person who initially finds their partner relaxing to be around may later get irritated by the slower, more lackadaisical style. They might grow weary of being the "spark plug" that gets the other going, saying to themselves, "What does it take to get you going? You feel like a dead weight! Come on, take some initiative!"

It's important to remember in these moments of frustration that our partner is modeling our opposite way of being. Instead of being annoyed, we can inquire within as to how we can become more balanced. We can be curious instead of critical about the other person's style, wondering how they manage to do that. If we can move a bit in their direction, our tendency to become annoyed will lessen, if not vanish.

Occasionally, people will match their charge to another. Two type A personalities may find commonality in their high-charge partner and may enjoy that they've finally found someone whose energy "matches." Two relaxed people may enjoy lounging around at home together, not doing much of anything. These relationships often have more harmony but tend to have a weaker spark between the two people. This may translate as less sexual charge, less intensity, and less challenge, but also less growth.

The Charge of Polarity: The Way to Keep Things Juicy

Corinne and Amanda were perplexed. They had been dating for about a year and had just moved in together. While they dated, they had a hot, steamy love life, but now that they were together under one roof, their passion had diminished. They were still in love, but they were now irritating each other, sparking into little fights that were creating distance. They missed the loving passion and wondered if it meant the relationship was doomed.

While most couples find resonance through what they have in common, it's actually *difference* that creates the strongest flow of charge between two people. If you want to keep your relationship alive and juicy, you must honor these differences, including the separations, misunderstandings, and each other's need for space and distance.

When we first find someone we think might be the love of our life (or for many, just a new relationship), most people want to merge. New lovers relish the discovery that the other person likes the same old movies, is an avid reader of Shakespeare, or loves to tango dance. Falling in love can be seen as a process of taking down boundaries and moving toward "becoming one."

That's all fine and dandy as an ideal, but a funny thing happens as you move in that direction: *the erotic charge diminishes.* For many couples, this is mysterious. Like Corinne and Amanda, they still feel the love, but they're no longer having that can't-get-enough-of-you feeling they had when they were first together. That's because they lost their differentiation.

David Schnarch, in his book *Passionate Marriage,*[2] describes the drive for individuality as equally important to the drive for togetherness. A healthy relationship needs to have a balance of both. If we lose our individuality, we lose our sense of self and fall prey to emotional fusion. We begin to live through the other person, who might be inwardly saying, "How can I miss you if you won't go away?"

In Greek mythology, Eros is an ancient god who represents the force of attraction, from which we get our word *erotic.* Eros is desire, in the form of arousal, lust, sexuality, and the simple urge to become close to someone. According to Freud, Eros was the force of life itself, strongly connected with libido, his word for charge. But Eros has a counterpart, Thanatos, the force of death or separation, who can appear as aggression, destruction, or even violence. The two brothers do a balancing act in the field of relationship. Much as we might like one better than the other, it's important to honor both and the endless dance between them.

While this is not a support of violence in relationship by any means, the little misunderstandings that result in "having our differences" create enough separation that Eros can then be renewed. When Eros is overindulged and we want to be close all the time, we are actually inviting Thanatos to create distance in a more extreme way, so that Eros doesn't burn out.

For Corinne and Amanda, it was Corinne who wanted to be close and Amanda who would then pull away, become grumpy, or even pick a fight. But once she closed off to her partner, she would miss her and Amanda would try to get back into her good graces and be close again. I assured them that it didn't mean their relationship was failing. Instead, I encouraged them to court Thanatos consciously, by asserting their boundaries and their need for time apart and by pursuing their own interests outside the relationship. As predicted, this enhanced their erotic connection.

One of the ways Thanatos can show up, however, is in the ways our partner can trigger us. Then we need to understand how charge plays out through these triggers.

Harville Hendrix, a well-known relationship guru, was once teaching a couples' workshop at a place where I was also teaching. Because I couldn't go to his workshop, we had lunch together, where I asked him, "Harville, if you were to distill down the main thing you are teaching these couples, what would it be?" He smiled and answered, "Know that you are in relationship with someone who is different than you are. Respect the differences, and don't try to make them the same." Good advice for keeping your relationship juicy and respectful at the same time.

Partners Trigger Each Other's Charge

If you have hidden pockets of charge—and we all do—it's inevitable that your partner will trigger it sooner or later. A simple word, phrase, or gesture may get you boiling or quaking in fear. Or perhaps you suddenly shut down, becoming sullen and withdrawn. Regardless of how you react, triggers offer an enormous opportunity for growth, *if* you can manage them with awareness and skill.

When you're triggered, your charge rises almost instantaneously. Unless you have a well-developed awareness, the heightened charge simply strengthens your defenses. Think of how entrenched someone becomes in his point of view during an argument. For someone who felt overly controlled as a child, just hearing a simple request from their partner might trigger a charge of anger and resistance. For another who may have been frequently criticized, such a request fuels the belief that they're not good enough, and the charge spirals down in a black pit of despair. For still another, their partner's sullen withdrawal triggers their fears of abandonment. Someone who falls into crying jags may trigger guilt and responsibility in their partner.

When you're triggered, the excess charge makes it difficult, if not impossible, to receive much of anything. Think of how hard it is to give someone a hug when they're angry or how difficult it is to get them to listen. Until discharge occurs, there is simply no room for new input. When your patterns get triggered, you literally *become* your patterns, rather than the essence of your true self.

You don't have a bad relationship because triggers occur. They arise in almost any long-term relationship, especially the ones where there are lessons to learn. Add kids and jobs and all the other things that couples (gay, straight, or otherwise) deal with, and voilà, the opportunity for triggers is magnified. The crux of a successful relationship lies in the ability to circumvent the trap of triggers that can spiral into destruction and instead maximize the healing they can bring.

I had the privilege at one time of working on these issues with my colleague and communications specialist, Susan Campbell, Ph.D. What follows is heavily drawn from her work and her excellent short book, co-authored with John Grey, *Five-Minute Relationship Repair*.[3] For further detail on the following process, I suggest getting this book. I have adapted her steps here and combined them with my own steps on working with charge. The result is an effective process you can use to turn a destructive cycle into empathy, awareness, and intimacy.

How to Handle Triggers in a Relationship

Step One: Take a Pause

The first step is to recognize that you're triggered and request a pause or time-out. This gives you a specific amount of time to disengage from the situation and feel your own charge. The time-out period could be 10 minutes or it could be a few hours, but it always includes an agreement to return to the issue after a specified amount of time. A person could say, "I need a time-out for fifteen minutes, and promise to come back at nine fifteen." Or you might say, "I'm really stressed from a tough day at work, and rather than dump all that on you, I need a couple of hours to wind down and get some dinner. Can we return to this discussion at eight thirty this evening after I've had something to eat and the kids have gone to bed?"

It's recommended to set up this agreement ahead of time—when you're not triggered—so you can just refer to it in the heat of the moment. Identify a key word or gesture that signifies "charge overload" and a need for some time-out. The agreement states that when one person asks for a pause, the other agrees to allow it to happen. It also states that it is *only* a pause, not an excuse to avoid the issues. I know from experience that I have hated it when my partner needs to pause while I'm in the heat of my emotions, but I have also learned that nothing will get accomplished in this state. Knowing—and then experiencing—that the issue will be picked up later helps to build trust in the process.

Step Two: Inner Reflection

Notice your charge. During the pause, take some time alone to reflect. Don't check your cell phone or e-mail. Don't watch TV or play a game on the computer. Instead, notice your charge and what it's doing. What are your body sensations? Where is the charge most concentrated? Where are you constricting against your charge? Where do you feel pressure or tension? What does the charge make you want to do? Do you need to discharge a little by making sound, pacing, or pushing on something? Do you need to self-soothe or comfort yourself?

Experience your charge fully, owning it and befriending it. If possible, write down your sensations and reflect upon them as part of your pattern. Consider them in terms of your character structure, your chakra imbalances, or any other blocks that you are aware of as described in the previous chapters.

Examine your emotions. Emotions usually have a repeating theme. One person may habitually go to sadness, another to fear, still another may be quick to anger. You might be prone to worry or dread, frequently feel hurt or lonely, or just get frustrated or go numb. Ask yourself when you have felt that way before, especially as a child. Were you angry when your brother picked on you? Were you sad when your mom didn't have time for you?

Examine your fears. Positive emotions are an attempt to move toward something; "negative" emotions are trying to avoid something. What are the core fears underneath your feelings? What are you trying to avoid? Are you afraid you will be abandoned, overwhelmed, controlled, trapped, used, helpless, or insignificant? Write down any words about what you are objecting to and the core fears behind your emotion. It doesn't matter if these fears are realistic, but that they are present. You may fear that your husband is going to leave you, even though consciously you know that is unlikely.

Examine your beliefs. What is the story you are telling yourself about the situation? Within that story is your set of beliefs. Move from the story to an inquiry of the beliefs that may be operating. If you tell yourself, "He never listens to me," notice if you have a belief that "no one listens to you," or that you're not worthy of being listened to. If you tell yourself, "It's useless. It will never work," notice if that is a belief that operates in other areas of your life. What do you believe about yourself that makes you powerless? Do you believe you will be punished if you take action? That you will fail? That you have no support? Simply become aware of these beliefs—and that they are only beliefs. They aren't necessarily true, even though we might find ample evidence to support them.

Identify your needs. Beneath our core fears lie hidden needs. Our fear is that these needs will not get met. More often, needs are not even acknowledged, so identifying them is a first step. Are you needing to feel connected? Respected? Valued? Supported? Wanted? Are you needing to know that someone is there for you, that you can count on them, that you can trust what you're told? State your needs in terms of your own process, rather than what the other person is doing. Instead of saying, "You never consider my feelings!" state your need as, "I have a need to hear that my feelings matter to you." "I need to know that you are still committed to being with me." "I have a need to feel that I matter . . . that I can speak up and be heard . . . that my boundaries are respected . . . that I am appreciated . . . that we are a team . . ."

Step Three: Return from Your Pause

Once you have done this inner work, you can return to your partner. Most likely you will feel more connected to yourself, to your truth, and to your needs. Acknowledge what triggered you and the behavior you exhibited. "I realize I got snarky and insulting when we were arguing." "I realize I blamed you for what I was feeling." "I can see that I got shut down and cold when I felt criticized." Then you can share the story you told yourself, along with your core feelings and fears. "I told myself you didn't love me anymore, that I could never do it right, that I would never please you. I felt hurt and betrayed." And then finally, state your needs: "What I really needed was to be reassured that we are connected and that I matter to you." "What I really needed was to ask for help, rather than criticize."

Then you can apologize for the reactive behavior and ask for a "do-over." You can say something like, "I'm really sorry I insulted you, and I would like to take it back. If I could do it over, I would let you know that I was feeling scared and vulnerable, and I would have been able to tell you I needed some reassurance that you weren't going to leave me."

Ideally, the partner can respond with an acknowledgment of the feelings and a reassuring gesture or statement. He or she might say, "Now I see how that really scared you, and I want to tell you how much I appreciate who you are and that you mean a great deal to me."

Once this process is complete with one person, the other can take a turn with the same process. In general, I would let the person who is most triggered go first, as long as the pause allowed their charge to come back down to a manageable level.

One of the gifts of intimate, long-term relationships is that it gives us a chance to see our patterns. Only by having them triggered over and over again can we recognize these patterns as something within ourselves and use that awareness to uncover key aspects of our psyche that need healing. If we can weather the storm and engage our partner in this process, we can harvest the charge and the insights and create greater intimacy and longevity.

chapter 25

CHARGE
and
SOCIETY

||||||||||||||||||||||||||||||||||||||||||||||||||||||||||||||||||||||

Things fall apart; the center cannot hold;
Mere anarchy is loosed upon the world,
The blood-dimmed tide is loosed, and everywhere
The ceremony of innocence is drowned;
The best lack all conviction, while the worst
Are full of passionate intensity.

WILLIAM BUTLER YEATS (1919)

Whether it's people attending a conference, a concert, a march, a political rally, a revival church service, a neighborhood meeting, or even a family gathering, *group charge* can be a powerful force. It can be the source of change or stagnation, creation or destruction. If our own charge is triggered or multiplied by combining it with another, how does that charge behave in larger groups?

You might even say the effectiveness of a group is directly related to how well the group can channel the charge of a bunch of individuals into a single purpose. The strength of the group, however, is not defined by whether that purpose is good or bad, for it can go either way. The Catholic Inquisition brutally burned hundreds of thousands of innocent women (and some men) accused of witchcraft. Hitler's Nazi Germany created catastrophic human rights abuses and the largest death toll of any war in history. The rogue group ISIS (Islamic State of Iraq and Syria) is a modern example of the way unhealed charge from the traumatization of war can create a violent force for terrorism.

Groups can also create benevolent change, as witnessed by the civil rights movement, peace marches, Black Lives Matter, the Occupy movement, women's rights, gay rights, and environmental protection. In fact, it seems to be the only way that major changes in values, politics, and society take place—through the successful motivation of group charge, focused on a particular issue.

We've talked about how, as individuals, we need to be able to run our charge through our core, to be in the center of our charge. This is equally true of a group. Does it have a coherent core of organization, values, and strategy? If not, as Yeats describes in the chapter-opening quote, the center cannot hold. When that happens, those with the most charge—the dispossessed, traumatized, and angry—will dominate the group with their "passionate intensity," while those with less charge lose heart and "all conviction." The result, as we have witnessed through history, can be disastrous. In a tinderbox world with nuclear weapons, teetering on the precipice of environmental collapse while subject to dictators and demagogues, understanding charge in groups is essential.

When values are rapidly changing—as they are in an increasingly globalized, technological, environmentally stressed, and overpopulated world, the center does not always hold. Values that once defined Western society—imperial domination, obedience to authority, competition over cooperation, profits before people and planet, and hierarchical structures that render individuals powerless—are no longer serving a dynamic, diverse, and radically more informed and empowered citizenry. The old center is shifting. It can no longer hold.

But new movements take time to form a coherent center. Their initial efforts can seem impotent, their messages confusing, their purpose conflicted. We're impatient with the process of consolidating new ideas. Even when the old forms no longer work, their ideas are at least familiar and often simpler than the more complex challenges of the new. The tendency to go "back to basics" in a time of uncertainty makes it even more difficult for the tender shoots of a new movement to take hold and find its power. Without respect for status quo, groups can lose cohesion. But too much adherence to the status quo makes the group stagnate.

The danger is this: the disowned charge of individuals can be harnessed by a powerful leader who acknowledges and directs that charge—even if the solutions proposed are damaging or unrealistic. Once the disowned charge is awakened and gets moving in a particular direction, it is extremely difficult to stop—as evidenced by Hitler and other malevolent dictators through history.

What is needed, now more than ever, is informed, effective leadership that rises up from the people to articulate and inspire a guiding vision of who we are and what we can become on this planet. A leader's message may be on point, but unless he or she can channel the charge of the group into meaningful and effective action, the message does not take hold. The center does not form.

Here's something to remember: *charge is not generated by the rational mind.* Facts and figures do not generate charge. Statistics on climate change, data on the gaps between rich and poor, reports of the number of innocent people killed in some suicide bombing—these things rarely motivate, even though we think they should. Instead, people are moved when they *feel* something, and their emotions move them to *do* something. A picture of one child, floating dead in the ocean, has more impact than statistics that tell us 65 million refugees walk the planet looking for a home. We simply relate to other humans more than numbers.

This was abundantly clear in the 2016 U.S. election. Both Bernie Sanders and Donald Trump were able to mobilize the charge in their followers into a collective movement. Both Trump and Sanders had messages that were relatively simple: *they basically stood against something and spoke to people's unacknowledged charge about the way things were going for them.* They stood against joblessness, exploitation, and corruption in government, even though their personalities, intentions, and solutions to these problems were hugely different. They skillfully tapped into the emotional charge of unexpressed anger and gave it a target. Despite other factors that may have influenced the election, Hillary Clinton's message, practical as it was, did not motivate enough group excitement to carry her safely over the finish line, even though the majority of people agreed with her policies.

Theories of Groups and Charge

Let's look at some of the ways groups handle charge, whether consciously or unconsciously, and what happens to an individual's charge in the process. There are several theories to consider, but let's start with Freud. As you know, Freud divided the personality into three components: the id, the ego, and superego, representing our unconscious impulses, our executive identity, and our conscience.

Freud postulated that the anonymity of being in crowds relaxes the hold of the superego, bringing the id's impulses closer to the surface. The crowd then provides a way to release these urges that would otherwise be repressed.[1] In other words, once you see someone smashing a window, the hidden desire to do the same thing surfaces and overpowers your restraint. You suddenly have permission to let out your feelings in a destructive act.

In the late nineteenth century, Gustave Le Bon described three main processes that occur in crowds: *submergence, contagion,* and *suggestion.*[2] In the first stage, submergence, a person loses their sense of a separate self in the anonymity of the crowd. The larger the crowd, the more anonymous an individual becomes. They can now get away with things that they might never do at work or at home. They can yell or scream, break windows or hurl insults, with far less personal responsibility.

As they come into contact with others (contagion) in a similar state, they are now more easily influenced, just as you are more likely to catch a contagious disease if your immune system is lowered. We simply become more susceptible through contact with others, especially when we have lost the sense of our individual self.

If suggestions are then inserted into the crowd, such as a politician at a political rally having the group chant something or an angry demonstrator throwing stones through windows, these ideas are more likely to be adopted without intellectual critique. The crowd becomes programmed by the suggestions and fueled by the emotional charge—without being aware that this is happening. Instead they *think* they are operating under individual choice, which is why people defend their views so vehemently when challenged by an outsider.

On the positive side, this can create an uplifting of spirit known as a group high. Consider the *kirtan,* an evening of call-and-response chanting, accompanied by a few instruments and drums. As the rhythm of the chants are repeated over and over again by performers and audience, the personal ego surrenders to the collective experience. We dissolve the illusion of separateness and feel the unity that is the essence of spiritual awakening. We become larger than our ordinary selves. This can also happen at concerts, raves, marches, and inspiring speeches.

On the negative side, we can be sold on ideas that go against our best interest and commit moral atrocities that cause irrevocable damage. The group high and the danger are not mutually exclusive. It depends on the ideas inserted into the fertile group mind.

George Lakoff, a political commentator and former linguistics professor at UC Berkeley, describes how 98 percent of our thought process is unconscious. Thoughts, however, have a physical reality in the neural circuitry in the brain, which is triggered largely by language. Repetitive phrases strengthen that circuitry, binding the neurons together and increasing the likelihood of that thought. We know this well from advertising that links repetitive phrases with catchy little tunes. It's equally true of speeches that repeat key phrases and political slogans. It can be used for good or ill. Martin Luther King and Donald Trump both employed the power of repetition.

This boils down to four main theories about how group energy forms, in which the following kinds of collective charge can be seen.

1. Convergence theory. Individuals enjoy coming together with like-minded others. They have a chosen interest or purpose prior to meeting but are then strengthened by others with the same interest. Examples are:

- *Conferences.* We know that it's not so much the speakers but the conversation in the hallways that make conferences so energizing. The subject could be computers, martial arts, alternative healing, cars, dogs, or yoga, but the interest is already present, then is enlivened by contact with others.

- *Sports games.* Attending a basketball, baseball, or football game and rooting for your side is an energizing experience. Individuals pick a side before attending, but in the course of the game they become charged up by the other fans in the stadium. Whether their side wins or loses the game influences whether their experience makes them feel triumphant or despondent.

2. **De-individuation theory.** Individuals have lost their own meaning and purpose, or they are stripped of their individuality, which is then repurposed by the goal of the group, for better or worse.

- *The military.* Upon being accepted into the military, one is shaved, given a uniform, and made to live with others whose beds, clothing, and behavior are all the same. Stripped of individuality, a person's energy is then channeled into the military goal, even to the point of risking one's life for a cause they might not believe in.

- *Neighborhood gangs, terrorists.* Unhealed trauma, destroyed hopes, and lack of individual identity can drive a person to join a gang or a rogue group like ISIS. Within the gang, they have a new, shared identity and will do whatever it takes, even commit horrendous crimes, in order to maintain their identity as a member of the group.

3. Emergent Norm Theory. This happens when a crowd has no purpose but someone emerges to give it one. That person could be a dictator or a benevolent leader or someone who emerges from the group itself.

- *Political rallies.* One might be unsure of their views but then influenced by the ideas of the leader or speaker.

- *Patriotism.* A disparate citizenry becomes fired up by a foreign threat. The massive influx of American flags after the 9/11 destruction of the World Trade Center in 2001 was a classic example. Wars invoke patriotism and channel disparate energy toward a single enemy or cause.

4. Social Identity Theory. Slightly different than the convergence theory that brings people together with common interests, this theory has more to do with prior identity.

- *Bigotry.* Social identity can increase bigotry, as one group strengthens their group identity at the cost of the other. Racism, sexism, homophobia, and xenophobia are all examples of social identity that is energized through seeing one's own group as superior to other groups. The polarities between "us" and "them" increases the charge and often the oppression.

- *Resistance to bigotry.* The reverse is also true. Groups finding common identity as women, Jews, Christians, Pagans, Native Americans, African Americans, or even Democrats, Republicans, or Green Party members, come together through common social identity to fight oppression of their group.

- *Religious persecution.* Similar to bigotry, the group identity carries the belief of moral superiority, supported by their interpretation of some religious doctrine, and is therefore justified in punishing or demeaning another group that is not of the same beliefs.

How to Maximize Group Energy

So how do we use this information to create positive change? How can the owning of our own charge help to organize and channel group energy consciously for the benefit of our world?

- *Awaken possibility.* Motivational speakers awaken a sense of possibility in their audience, lifting them out of their limitations and promising some kind of reward. If their techniques work, this can be a great service; when they don't, it can be disappointing, if not downright manipulative. Most of these techniques require follow-through in the participants, so the speaker must get them charged up enough to take action after the talk.

- *Speak to pain or fear.* We all have pain, whether it's emotional, financial, physical, or relational. Most of it goes unnoticed, but tremendous charge can be awakened when the pain is addressed and solutions offered. Stories are the best way to accomplish this, as they engage the listener on an emotional level.

- *Highlight the goals that motivate.* We are goal-oriented creatures. People get charged up when there's something valuable at stake. The Gold Rush motivated people to move westward. Values motivate people through religions and politics. Needs motivate groups such as the Occupy movement or Black Lives Matter.

- *Empowerment.* When people are empowered to be themselves, to make change, or to rise above oppression, they join forces with others of like mind and heart. The feminist, civil rights, and gay movements have found empowerment through groups energized to fight oppression.

- *Novelty.* What inspires something to go viral on YouTube? Novelty. What inspires people to buy a new product? Novelty makes something remarkable, which means people will remark about it and spread it through word of mouth.

- *Humor and pleasure.* Comedians have great command of their audiences, and it's all done through pleasure and enjoyment. Performers and beautiful stage sets delight their audiences. People are always drawn toward pleasure and enjoyment, especially in times of stress and uncertainty. Political satirists are a major source of news for many people.

Ultimately, we join groups because it charges us up. We get energized by others, and we bring that charge home. As we reclaim our own charge, we are less likely to be manipulated by others and more likely to be able to consciously join together in groups for a positive cause and not be so weak that we get swept up without questioning, into questionable behaviors.

When we own our charge within and join together with others toward a common purpose, we can change the world.

chapter 26

CONCLUSION

|||||||||||||||||||||||||||||||||||||||||||||||||||||||||||||||||||||||||||||||||||||||||||

LIVING A FULL-CHARGE LIFE

Energy is the living, vibrating ground of your being, and it is your body's natural self-healing elixir, its natural medicine.

DONNA EDEN

I love those moments at the end of a workshop when everyone is glowing. I look out at the faces and remember how during the week, each one turned on at different moments, like flowers blooming in a garden. New possibilities have opened up. I myself am energized by it, even though I know I'll crash into a puddle of exhaustion an hour later. Such is the ebb and flow of charge.

I also love those moments alone with a client when they are in their full charge—even if it's a cascade of tears, a fiery rage, or just that clear and present look in the eyes when someone is deeply in touch with their true self. The energy that emanates from the being in front of me fills the room. I know I am in the presence of the Divine. It makes my work holy.

It's a gift to be with someone in their full charge. Though many of us were taught being in our fullness would diminish someone else, I find the truth is just the opposite. We invite others to come alive when we ourselves are alive. We *want* to be full of ourselves and to be with others who are also full of themselves. Being full of yourself is not narcissism. When you're in touch with who you really are, you don't need others to affirm you.

However, it's not just about making our charge as big as possible. It's not a gift when our charge isn't grounded. It's not a gift when we unconsciously discharge our emotions on other people, and it's certainly not a gift when a parent does that to a child.

And it might not feel like a gift in those moments when we're streaming with the emotion of a past hurt. It doesn't feel like a gift when we are locked down against our charge, frozen in trauma, or bound up in ways we feel powerless to change. Yet these experiences are all steps to healing and reclaiming our aliveness.

Ultimately, energy wants to be free, but it's not a wild and crazy freedom; it's not chaotic and scattered. Too much freedom without a balance of containment doesn't concentrate the charge. It dissipates in aimlessness and doesn't become power. But too much containment blocks the charge and doesn't let it complete its journey. When we're bound up, our charge isn't available to us—at least not in a way that's useful.

The Journey

We're all on a journey. As we travel, we want the highways to be clear and free so we can drive without traffic jams or roadblocks. But we don't drive just anywhere we want—we follow the lines and signs on the road, flowing with traffic, not against it. We flow with the energy, and it takes us to our destination. The journey is its own destination. When we reach completion of any part of it, there is an "Ah" factor. Satisfied, we rest, until it becomes time to journey again.

We take this journey through the vehicle of our body. The body is equipped with just about everything you need for the journey, but it does require fuel and someone to drive it. Awareness is the driver of the vehicle. It decides where to go and when to speed up or slow down, and it knows how to adjust the steering wheel for subtle changes in the road. But awareness is not separate from the body. It is anchored in it. You can't drive your car from outside the vehicle; you must be in the driver's seat.

Driving the vehicle requires not only consciousness but energy—a constant and steady supply of it. We want to be able to tap that energy appropriately—to go fast when the coast is clear and to slow down for more difficult terrain. We want enough energy to get us to the next destination, the next point of rest, a place where we can recharge. We want to use the right kind of fuel and keep the body in good repair so it doesn't require more energy than necessary.

The chakras can be seen as a map for the journey. Understanding how charge flows through each chakra can help you navigate life's twists and turns to better go where you want to go. But chakras also act as resistors and capacitors—they speed energy up or slow it down, depending on what's needed or blocked. Clearing and balancing your chakras keeps the gears of your vehicle moving as you shift from one mode to another.

Our character structure is the kind of vehicle we're in. We're a station wagon or a sports car. We ride a bicycle or drive a flatbed truck. Each one handles energy differently and has its own advantages and drawbacks. A sports car looks good but isn't very practical. A bicycle is nice and light, open to the air and scenery, but it can't carry much. A truck is sturdy but takes a lot of energy to get it going. The only difference here is that our character structure can change over time. We can expand or lighten up, firm up the body or soften it.

Along the journey, we need the freedom to be who we are. We need to be able to choose the nature of our travel and our attitude toward it. We need others to journey with us, to share in the joys and sorrows along the way. The questions we can't answer right away beckon us to look deeper into the mystery. Ideally the journey is full of discovery—and never ends.

Humanity is on a journey as well. I believe our evolutionary journey is to realize our divine potential. We are here to heal and awaken ourselves, to guide the healing and awakening of others along the way, and to create a glorious world that our great-great-grandchildren can treasure. I call that world "heaven on earth."

There are incredible challenges facing humanity at this time as we journey from what I call the "love of power" to the "power of love."[1] We live in an automated world in which power and authority are seen as outside of us, rather than within. Our love of power has come from our own powerlessness, which is a disconnection from our own charge. If there is any silver lining to oppression, it is the way it forces us to awaken our individual and collective power. To rise up to freedom, we must awaken the charge within us and learn to channel that charge into productive activity, not just alone but together with others.

A society of free individuals—awake to their aliveness, in touch with their own charge—can take humanity in a new direction. People in their full charge cannot easily be subdued or manipulated. They do not ruthlessly consume everything around them. They are not trying to fill an emptiness that comes from disconnection with the self. They are not trying to be like everyone else. They are each a unique expression of the Divine.

A society of free individuals has its own challenges. How do we work together? How do we listen to one another and forge a world that truly works? We begin by making sure each part works well within itself, then in its intimate relationships, and finally combining with others through groups.

The overarching reason to harvest your charge is to live your life to the fullest extent possible—to live fully into everything you do, to enjoy each moment, even the challenges. Our aliveness is our birthright. It is glorious when we can embrace it fully and come together with others who are doing the same.

And when that happens, anything can be accomplished!

Additional Resources

Books by Anodea Judith

Chakras: Seven Keys to Awakening and Healing the Energy Body (Carlsbad, CA: Hay House, 2016).

Anodea Judith's Chakra Yoga (St. Paul, MN: Llewellyn Publications, 2015).

Creating on Purpose: The Spiritual Technology for Manifesting through the Chakras, co-authored with Lion Goodman (Boulder, CO: Sounds True, 2012).

Eastern Body, Western Mind: Psychology and the Chakra System as a Path to the Self (Berkeley, CA: Celestial Arts, 1997).

Wheels of Life: A User's Guide to the Chakra System, revised (St. Paul, MN: Llewellyn Publications, 1987, 1999).

Chakra Balancing (Boulder, CO: Sounds True, 2003).

The Global Heart Awakens: Humanity's Rite of Passage from the Love of Power to the Power of Love (San Rafael, CA: Shift Books, 2013).

Other Energy-Healing Books

Ann Adams and Karin Davidson, *EFT Level 1 Comprehensive Training Resource* (Fulton, CA: Energy Psychology Press, 2011).

Susan Campbell and John Grey, *Five-Minute Relationship Repair: Quickly Heal Upsets, Deepen Intimacy, and Use Differences to Strengthen Love* (Novato, CA: New World Library, 2015).

Donna Eden, *Energy Medicine: Balancing Your Body's Energies for Optimal Health, Joy, and Vitality* (New York: Penguin Books, 1998, 2008).

David Feinstein and Donna Eden, *The Promise of Energy Psychology: Revolutionary Tools for Dramatic Personal Change* (New York: Penguin Books, 2005).

Stanley Keleman, *Emotional Anatomy* (Berkeley, CA: Center Press, 1985.)

Steven Kessler, *The 5 Personality Patterns: Your Guide to Understanding Yourself and Others and Developing Emotional Maturity* (Richmond, CA: Bodhi Tree Press, 2015).

Peter A. Levine, *In an Unspoken Voice: How the Body Releases Trauma and Restores Goodness* (Berkeley, CA: North Atlantic Books, 2010).

Alexander Lowen, M.D., *Bioenergetics: The Revolutionary Therapy That Uses the Language of the Body to Heal the Problems of the Mind* (New York: Penguin Books/Arkana, 1975).

John Pierrakos, *Core Energetics: Developing the Capacity to Love and Heal* (Mendocino, CA: Life Rhythm Publication, 1987).

Recommended Websites

Association for Comprehensive Energy Psychology: www.energypsych.org

HeartMath Institute: www.heartmath.org

Somatic Experiencing trainings and practitioners: www.traumahealing.org

United States Association for Body Psychotherapy: www.usabp.org

Belief work: www.clearyourbeliefs.com

Author's websites: www.AnodeaJudith.com, www.SacredCenters.com

Donna Eden's Energy Medicine: www.learnenergymedicine.com

Endnotes

Chapter 4

1. Jessie Carney Smith and Linda T. Wynn, *Freedom Facts and Figures: 400 Years of African American Civil Rights Expression* (Conton, MI: Visible Ink Press, 2009), 35.
2. Ibid., 58.
3. George Leonard, *The Silent Pulse: A Search for the Perfect Rhythm that Exists in Each of Us* (Layton, UT: Gibbs Smith, 2006), 116–18.

Chapter 5

1. Stanley Keleman, *Embodying Experience: Forming a Personal Life* (Berkeley, CA: Center Press, 1987), 9.

Chapter 7

1. John Pierrakos, *Core Energetics: Developing the Capacity to Love and Heal* (Mendocino, CA: Life Rhythm Publication, 1987), 26.

Chapter 8

1. Ann Adams and Karin Davidson, *EFT Level 1 Comprehensive Training Resource* (Fulton, CA: Energy Psychology Press, 2011).
2. David Feinstein, Ph.D., "Acupoint Stimulation in Treating Psychological Disorders: Evidence of Efficacy" (abstract), *Review of General Psychology* (2012). http://www.innersource.net/ep/images/stories/downloads/Acupoint_Stimulation_Research_Review.pdf

Chapter 9

1. Peter Levine, *Healing Trauma: Restoring the Wisdom of the Body* (Boulder, CO: Sounds True, 2012), 9.
2. Stephen Porges, "The Polyvagal Perspective" (abstract). http://stephenporges.com/index.php/scientific-articles/scientific-articles/publicationss/3-the-polyvagal-perspective.

Chapter 12

1. James W. Prescott, "Body Pleasure and the Origins of Violence," *The Bulletin of the Atomic Scientists* (November 1975): 10–20. http://www.violence.de/prescott/bulletin/article.html.

Chapter 13

1. National Institute of Mental Health: http://www.nimh.nih.gov/health/statistics/prevalence/any-anxiety-disorder-among-adults.shtml.

2. Depression and Bipolar Support Alliance: http://www.dbsalliance.org/site/PageServer?pagename=education_statistics_depression.

3. World Health Organization: http://www.who.int/mediacentre/factsheets/fs369/en/.

4. Alexander Lowen, M.D., *Bioenergetics: The Revolutionary Therapy That Uses the Language of the Body to Heal the Problems of the Mind* (New York: Penguin Books/Arkana, 1975), 47.

5. Donna Eden with David Feinstein, *Energy Medicine: Balancing Your Body's Energies for Optimal Health, Joy, and Vitality* (New York: Tarcher, 1998, 2008), 59.

6. Alex Korb, *The Upward Spiral: Using Neuroscience to Reverse the Course of Depression One Small Change at a Time* (Oakland, CA: New Harbinger Publications, 2015).

7. For more on how to change beliefs, see Anodea Judith and Lion Goodman's book: *Creating on Purpose: The Spiritual Technology of Manifesting through the Chakras* (Boulder, CO: Sounds True, 2012). Also see Lion Goodman's website: www.transformyourbeliefs.com.

8. For more tips on the psychological aspects of third chakra and family power dynamics, see Anodea Judith, *Eastern Body, Western Mind: Psychology and the Chakra System as a Path to the Self* (Berkeley, CA: Celestial Arts, 1996, 2004).

Chapter 14

1. L. Lanteaume, et al., "Emotion induction after direct intracerebral stimulations of human amygdala," *Cerebral Cortex* 17, no. 6 (July 2007): 1307–13. doi:10.1093/cercor/bhl041. PMID 16880223.

2. Neil R. Carlson, *Physiology of Behavior*, 11th ed. (London: Pearson, 2012), 608.

3. Daniel Goleman, *Emotional Intelligence: Why It Can Matter More Than IQ* (New York: Bantam, 1995), 24–26.

4. Doc Childre, Howard Martin, Deborah Rozman, and Rollin McCraty, *Heart Intelligence: Connecting with the Intuitive Guidance of the Heart* (Canada: Waterfront Press, 2016), 83.

5. Ibid., 79.

Chapter 15

1. Stephen R. Covey, *The 7 Habits of Highly Effective People: Powerful Lessons in Personal Change* (New York: Simon & Schuster, 1989), 247.

Chapter 19

1. Steven Kessler, *The 5 Personality Patterns: Your Guide to Understanding Yourself and Others and Developing Emotional Maturity* (Richmond, CA: Bodhi Tree Press, 2015).

Chapter 24

1. See Larry Dossey, M.D., *Prayer Is Good Medicine* (San Francisco, CA: Harper, 1994), or Larry Dossey, M.D., *Prayer Is Good Medicine: How to Reap the Healing Benefits of Prayer* (San Francisco, CA: Harper, 1997).

2. David Schnarch, *The Passionate Marriage: Keeping Love and Intimacy Alive in Committed Relationships* (New York: Beaufort Books, 1997).

3. Susan Campbell, Ph.D., and John Grey, *Five-Minute Relationship Repair: Quickly Heal Upsets, Deepen Intimacy, and Use Differences to Strengthen Love* (Novato, CA: New World Library, 2015).

Chapter 25

1. Sigmund Freud, *Group Psychology and the Analysis of the Ego* (New York: Sensory Press, 1921).

2. Gustav Le Bon, *The Crowd: A Study of the Popular Mind* (New York: Macmillan, 1896).

Chapter 26

1. For more on this, see Anodea Judith, *The Global Heart Awakens: Humanity's Rite of Passage from the Love of Power to the Power of Love* (San Rafael, CA: Shift Books, 2013).

Index

E

Earth. *See* Chakra one (earth)
Earth Skiing exercise, 234
Eating, 25
Eden, Donna, 152, *153*
Emergent norm theory, 289
Emotion
chakra one for, 130–137
charge accompanying, 6–7
for charging, 25–26
signs of too much or too little charge, 69–70
Emotional Freedom Technique (EFT), 82, 85–89. *See also* Tapping
Emotional Intelligence (Goleman), 169
Empathy. *See* Oral character structure
Encounter groups, 33–35
Endurer character structure, 235–246
charge pattern of, 239–241
example of, 235–237, *239*
gifts of, 241–242
healing for, 243–244
overview, 212–213
recognizing pattern of, 241
Tug-of-War exercise, 245
Will exercise, 245–246
wounding source of, 237–238
Energy. *See also* Charge
chakras as system of, 106–110, *107, 111*
charge definition and, 3–4
generating, 151–152
journey of, 294–296
mastery of, 144–145
maximizing group energy, 290–291
overlapping fields of, in relationships, 273
Energy Medicine (Eden), 152
Energy psychology (EP), 81–83. *See also* Tapping
Eros, 276–277
Esalen, 33–35
Exaggeration
awareness and exaggerating block, 66

Focus and Exaggerate exercise, 51–52
Exercise (physical activity)
for anxiety and depression, 147
charging or discharging with, 28, 30
Exercises
Alternate Nostril Breathing, 166
Authentic Movement exercise, 267
Boundary, 233–234
Breath of Fire, 154
Butterfly, 142
charging and discharging, 32
Charging Your Hand Chakras, 7
Cross Crawl, 152
Develop the Witness, 188–189
Doorway Push, 148
Earth Skiing, 234
Focus and Exaggerate, 51–52
Get off My Back, 179–180
HeartMath's Freeze-Frame Process, 169
Opening Leg Channels, 124–125
Pelvic Wave, 141–142
Pressing on the Jaw, 180
Punch Out, 154
Reflection (balance), 32
Reflection (chakra three), 155
Reflection (Challenger-Defender character structure), 255
Reflection (charge-discharge cycle), 41
Reflection (mind and body), 19
Reflection (Rigid character structure), 266
Schizoid Expansion, 226
Softening Meditation, 162–163
Stand Up and Shake, 148
Three Thumps, 152, *153*
Tug-of-War, 245
Twisting Breath, 165–166
Will, 245–246
Winged Breath, 165
Woodchopper, 148–149
Exercising your brain, 155–156
Exhaling, for discharging, 27

L

Lakoff, George, 287
Leaving Pattern, 221
Le Bon, Gustave, 286
Legs
  as discharge pathway, *71*, 72
  Opening Leg Channels, overview, 123–124
  Opening Leg Channels exercise, 124–125
  as roots of spine, 122–123
Leonard, George, 33–35
Levine, Peter, 92, 94
Life force. *See also* Awareness
  awareness of charge and, 64
  learning to master, 78–79
Light. *See* Chakra six (light)
Limbic resonance, 135
Love. *See* Chakra four (air)
Lover, 231. *See also* Oral character structure
Lowen, Alexander, 150

M

Masochist. *See* Endurer character structure
Massage, 30
Meaning, finding, 26
Meditation, 22, 29
Memories, 26–27
Memory, 185–186, 190–191
Meridians, 81, 83–85, *84*
Mind and body, 13–19. *See also* Chakra theory; Self-regulation; *individual chakras*
  interface for, 13–16
  as operating system, 16–17
  psychological complexes and charge, 17–18
  Reflection exercise for, 19

N

Negative charge, 8–9
Nervous system
  GABA (gamma-Aminobutyric acid), 147
  parasympathetic nervous system, 22
  sympathetic nervous system, 121–122
  synapses in, 129
Neurons, 187
Notice impulse, for awareness, 65

O

Operating system, mind and body as, 16–17
Oral character structure, 227–234
  Boundary exercise, 233–234
  charge pattern of, 230–231
  Earth Skiing exercise, 234
  example of, 227–228, *230*
  gifts of, 232
  healing for, 232–233
  overview, 212–213
  recognizing pattern of, 231
  wounding source of, 228–229
Orgasm, 28, 139–140
Outer charge, balancing inner charge with, 57–60
Outer compliance and inner defiance pattern, 150, 240
Overbinding, 56–57
Overcharging. *See also* Tapping
  awareness of, 69–70
  defined, 31–32

P

Parasympathetic nervous system, 22
Passionate Marriage (Schnarch), 276
Past experiences, chakra two and, 132–134
Pathways for discharging, *71*, 71–74
Pathways of charge, for trauma, 95–97
Pause
  for handling triggers in relationships, 279, 281–282
  pause and notice for awareness, 65
Pelvic Wave exercise, 141–142
Personality, Freud on, 286
Personal levels of comfort, 46–47, *47*
Physical sensations of charge, 5–7
Pierrakos, John, 78

Acknowledgments

As always, I am deeply grateful for the many unseen hands that go into writing and producing a book. First of all, I would like to honor my students and clients who taught me so much while I was teaching you. I developed this material over many years of work with you—thank you for your patience.

I would like to thank my teachers, some of whom I studied with directly, and others through their body of work: Peter Levine, Stanley Keleman, Alexander Lowen, John Pierrakos, and Cornelia and Siegmar Gerken.

I would like to acknowledge Shanon Dean, who created the charts and illustrations, to say nothing of her many years of support producing my websites, graphics, marketing, and general outreach. Gianna Carini also assists me in many tasks and gives me more time to do what I love, which is write.

I would like to thank Sally Mason-Swaab for her wonderful editing, and all the others at Hay House that have been part of this book: Reid Tracy, for seeing its value; the typesetter, Riann Bender; the proofreader, Andrea Monagle; the indexer, Joan Shapiro; and the graphic artist who did the cover design, Barbara LeVan Fisher.

And finally, I would like to thank my readers, for your willingness to learn something new, and your dedication to the healing process.

Anodea Judith
January, 2018

About the Author

Anodea Judith, Ph.D., is the author or co-author of eight books on various aspects of healing, psychology, spirituality, social change, and yoga, most notably as seen through the system of energy centers known as chakras. Her first book, released in 1987, *Wheels of Life*, has sold more than 250,000 copies in the U.S., with translations in 24 languages, selling even better today after nearly 30 years. She holds master's and doctoral degrees in psychology and human health, is a 500-hour registered yoga teacher (E-RYT), with lifelong studies of psychology, mythology, sociology, history, systems theory, and mystic spirituality. She is considered one of the country's foremost experts on the combination of chakras and therapeutic issues and on the interpretation of the chakra system for the Western lifestyle. She teaches across the world and has been a speaker at numerous conferences, and she is an ongoing faculty member of The Shift Network, Kripalu Yoga Center, New York Open Center, Omega, and many other retreat centers and yoga studios.

Website: www.anodeajudith.com

Hay House Titles of Related Interest

YOU CAN HEAL YOUR LIFE, the movie,
starring Louise Hay & Friends
(available as an online streaming video)
www.hayhouse.com/louise-movie

THE SHIFT, the movie,
starring Dr. Wayne W. Dyer
(available as an online streaming video)
www.hayhouse.com/the-shift-movie

———

CORE LIGHT HEALING:
My Personal Journey and Advanced Healing Concepts for
Creating the Life You Long to Live, by Barbara Ann Brennan

ENERGY STRANDS:
The Ultimate Guide to Clearing the Cords That Are
Constricting Your Life, by Denise Linn

REIKI:
Heal Your Body and Your Life with the Power
of Universal Energy, by Torsten A. Lange

THETAHEALING:
Introducing an Extraordinary Energy Healing Modality,
by Vianna Stibal

All of the above are available at your local bookstore,
or may be ordered by contacting Hay House (see next page).

———

We hope you enjoyed this Hay House book. If you'd like to receive our online catalog featuring additional information on Hay House books and products, or if you'd like to find out more about the Hay Foundation, please contact:

Hay House LLC, P.O. Box 5100, Carlsbad, CA 92018-5100
(760) 431-7695 or (800) 654-5126
(760) 431-6948 (fax) or (800) 650-5115 (fax)
www.hayhouse.com® • www.hayfoundation.org

———

Published in Australia by: Hay House Australia Pty. Ltd.,
18/36 Ralph St., Alexandria NSW 2015
Phone: 612-9669-4299 • *Fax:* 612-9669-4144
www.hayhouse.com.au

Published in the United Kingdom by: Hay House UK, Ltd.,
The Sixth Floor, Watson House, 54 Baker Street, London W1U 7BU
Phone: +44 (0)20 3927 7290 • *Fax:* +44 (0)20 3927 7291
www.hayhouse.co.uk

Published in India by: Hay House Publishers India,
Muskaan Complex, Plot No. 3, B-2, Vasant Kunj, New Delhi 110 070
Phone: 91-11-4176-1620 • *Fax:* 91-11-4176-1630
www.hayhouse.co.in

———

Access New Knowledge.
Anytime. Anywhere.

Learn and evolve at your own pace
with the world's leading experts.

www.hayhouseU.com

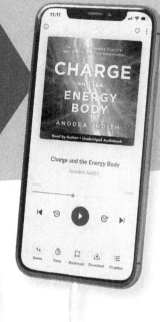